HOW TO EAT
Nutritional Strategies
To Unveil Your True Potential

Ryall Graber

Food Photography by: Malu Valencia
Cover Photography by: Moni Gonzalez
Additional Photography:
Carlos Loyo
Andras Schram
Renee Oliver
Book Design: Susan Vasconcelos
Chef: Oskar Rios

To my daughter Zuri.
May how I eat, how I live and how I love show you the way to achieving a lifetime of well-being.

To my parents, Linda and Dennis and my sister, Regan.
Thank you for believing in me and my crazy dreams, from the very beginning. Your continued love and support on my journey has enabled me to help thousands of people achieve their health and wellness goals - and more to come.

To my love, Marcelo.
Thank you for being the person who doesn't let their partner settle for less than they can achieve… This is real love. So grateful for all of the recipe testing and creating, the continued support and sacrifice you've made over the years to help me bring this book to life.

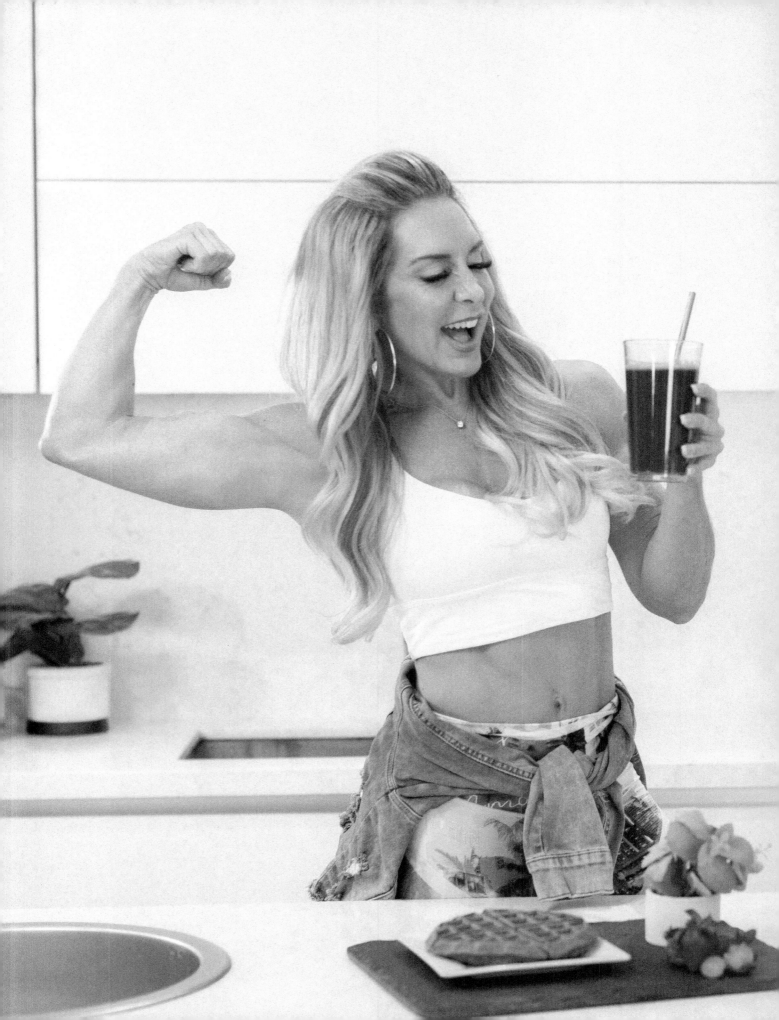

Table of Contents

Gain an improved understanding of the basic principles of nutrition and energy requirements while learning my top strategies for successful shopping, meal planning, all things healthy cooking, overcoming calorie counting, eating more intuitively and improving your relationship with food. Create your winning nutrition plan with this foundation.

Become an informed food master and overcome nutritional confusion on sugar, salt, water, alcohol, dairy, gluten, protein powder, misleading food labels, and organic foods. Get my tips on balancing your hormones with food, preventing disease with color, the garbage foods you want to kick and superfoods you want to pick to help you achieve optimal vitality. This chapter will set you straight— say 'hola' to feeling and looking your best.

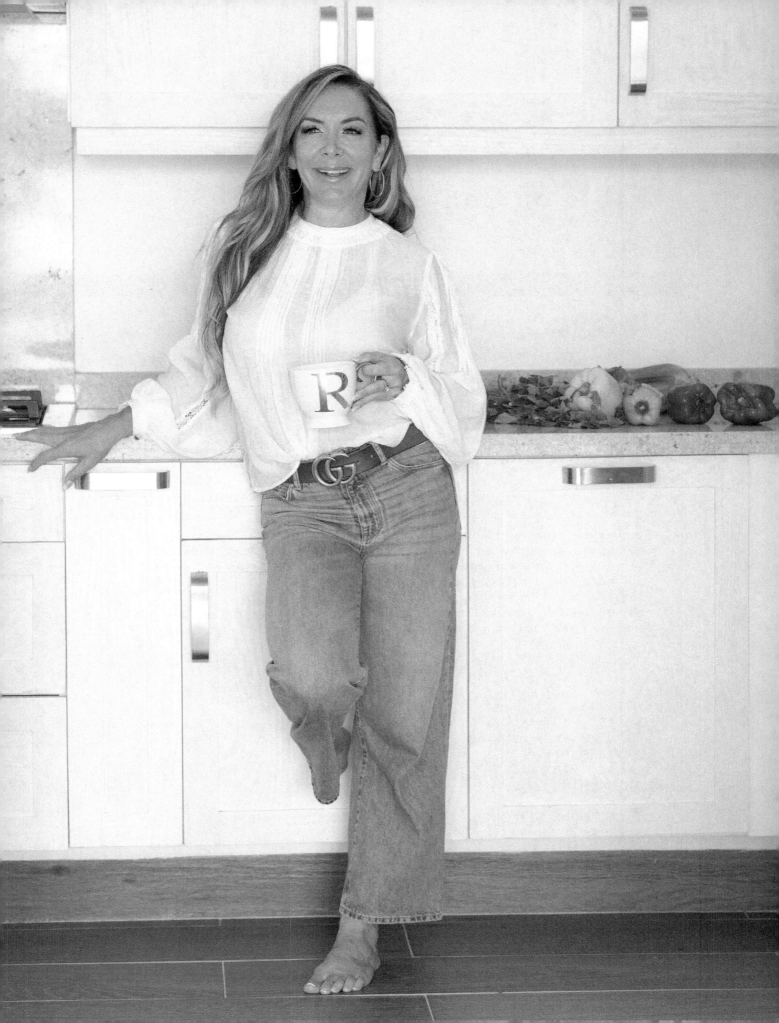

WELCOME, GORGEOUS!

Congratulations on buying my book—you've already made a commitment to change and you're on the path to a healthier life. I'm so proud of you! And I'm so happy you're joining me on this journey. How To Eat is your ultimate guide to living a vibrant and healthy life through food. The 120+ delicious and nutritious recipes combined with the knowledge, tips, and strategies I've learned over the past two decades, through trial and triumph, are going to change your life for the better. Say goodbye to nutritional confusion and yo-yo dieting. Say hello to feeling awesome, activating on your highest potential, food freedom and sailing through your days with ease. What is on the end of your fork is the answer, my friends. I've learned that food truly does have the power to revitalize our bodies at the highest level.

This book has something just for YOU! But before you dive in, it's important to know how to get the most out of this experience—which starts by knowing what your purpose is for reading this book.

If you're just looking for the recipes and aren't too interested in the learning aspect, then you're going to want to jump to the second half of the book. This is where you'll find all my bad-ass, delicious recipes that I've meticulously crafted on my quest to reach the top as a professional athlete while overcoming disordered eating, followed by years of fine-tuning to help my clients reach their highest potential. These recipes are the real deal and what you've been waiting for; they're simple to make, satiating, nutrient-dense, calorie-smart and delicious (I don't compromise on flavor and satisfaction!). You'll see the nutrition facts listed for each recipe; which have been calculated with the help of an online calculator and show estimated values. We aren't calorie counters here, but I have provided this for interest's sake. My hope for you is to worry less about the calories and more about the nutritional quality of the foods you're eating (hint: you may want to read the front section!).

If you're someone who wants brain food (AKA Knowledge) and wants to learn more about nutrition principles to optimize your life, then I suggest you start right from the beginning of the book. Read slowly and stop and reflect on all the information from the book to understand how the ideas can apply to you. Taking notes, highlighting, writing down ideas, and using page-markers to quickly reference pages will help you read the book more actively, not passively. By the time you get to the recipes, you'll be ready and eager to take action and apply your newfound food knowledge and start trying the recipes. And if you want to take it to the next level, see faster results and save time on menu planning, head over to my online shop and grab a goal-focused meal plan that uses the recipes in this book (https://ryallgraber.com/shop).

Now we're going to go deep; I've left no stone unturned, and I can't wait for you to experience this goodness. You'll find science-based information, written in a way that anyone can understand, fused with my experiences as an athlete, a coach, a recovered binge-eater, a food lover, a Mom, and an every-day, wanna-be superhero.

There is so much information and misinformation out there that it's difficult to know where to start. I want this book to be a place for you to start and a place to give you renewed hope. A place for you to feel empowered and finally say goodbye to dieting, to make simple, fun, delicious and nourishing meals while mastering how to eat, for yourself.

My most successful clients have always been action takers—for you to achieve the same results you have to put the tools and strategies in this book to work. Start making small changes from what you've learned in this book to build momentum. Stay consistent and connected to yourself. Step away from the scale; that little metal machine isn't allowed to determine your happiness or worth. Do more of what's making you feel good and less of what isn't. I promise you that these simple steps will lead to profound change. You're going to start to figure out what works best for you and your unique body. Establishing your own dietary lifestyle takes time and a willingness to try new foods, tastes, textures and flavors. Start by picking a few recipes and build on them every week. Before you know it you'll have twenty of your favorites that you can whip up without even looking at a recipe. The benefits of these recipes will start to speak for themselves. You'll start to feel better, and you'll start to look better.

Remember my friend, this is a lifestyle, not a diet. And achieving optimal vitality is an active pursuit, every single day. That's why I call it a 'wellness journey' as you must stay committed and practice your new found knowledge on a daily basis to attain the physical and mental health outcomes that you desire. You're also human, and life presents a series of endless distractions that will cause you to get off track or stall your progress. Don't feel guilty or beat yourself up when this happens, just get back on track with your healthy choices as soon as possible and remember why you want to live this lifestyle. Everyone gets distracted. In many ways, the real divide is between those who get back on track quickly and those who let interruptions expand into longer periods of inactivity. Top performers (I teach all of my clients to become champions!) get back on track faster than most. This is the skill you can develop. You will be interrupted, that is certain, but you can choose to keep it brief, reflect on it and move forward and re-align with your goals. If you want to change more than you want to stay the same, stay steadfast and focussed on what you want most. I'm confident that the information and recipes in this book will propel you to change your life for the better. If you want to change more than you want to stay the same, stay steadfast and focussed on what you want most.

I'm confident that the information and recipes in this book will propel you to change your life for the better. And, if you love the changes you're experiencing and want to further elevate, I invite you to either schedule an e-consult with me or apply to work with me 1x1 www.ryallgraber.com. My Transformation Coaching will help you unveil your 'inner champion' and achieve your highest goals. My superpower is helping people unlock their potential!

I'm so excited and honored to give you an in-depth look at my why and how I do what I do, and finally, to share my recipes, which I know people have been waiting several years for me to do. Thank you for being so patient and supporting my work. It's my hope that you feel it was well worth the wait. I can't wait to see your creations—tag me on social media @ryallwellness and use the hashtag #HowToEatTheBook. I'll be running giveaways and contests with some awesome prizes.

May this book enrich your life on every level. I'm so excited for your healthy and bright future.

Happy reading!

Ryall

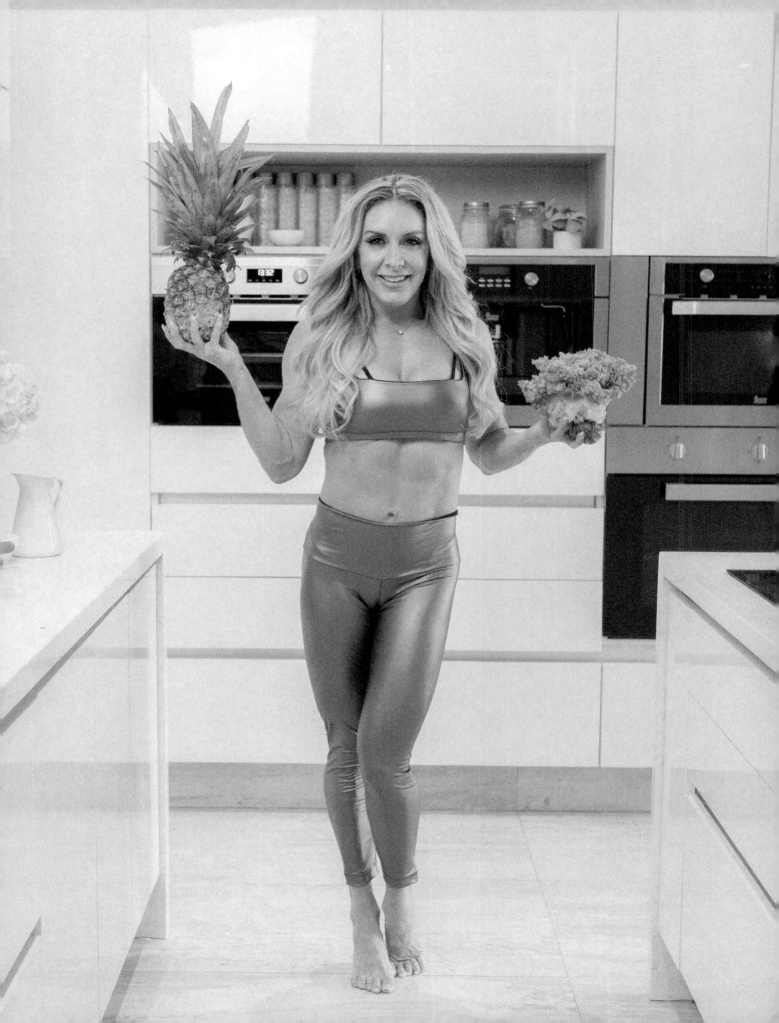

HOW IT ALL STARTED

I've always been a lover of food. Growing up in a small town in Alberta, Canada as an athletic child who loved gymnastics, skiing, and volleyball, I learned that food was essential for energy and recovery from a very young age. My parents were both competitive ice curlers (a massive sport in Canada); my father played at a national level—my childhood was submersed in sport, and I lived a very active lifestyle.

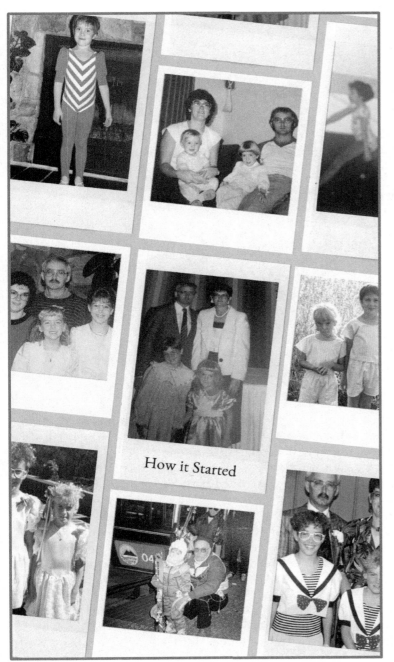

How it Started

Although my mother worked full-time, she was committed to preparing nourishing meals for my father, sister, and me. She would take my sister and me to the local farmers' market to shop for fresh foods in the summer. Family dinners were a daily occurrence and a priority, a time to eat, talk and connect. Like most Albertans, I grew up a 'steak and potatoes' kid. It was common to have hearty meals with bread and potatoes followed, on many occasions, by a delicious dessert. We were always encouraged not to take too much food; we had to 'clean our plates.' We didn't think much about health and disease, we didn't discuss what we should or shouldn't eat, and we didn't speak of diets and restrictions. We simply ate food that nourished us—we ate it together as a family, with gratitude. The fondest memories I have from my childhood are family gatherings over the holidays where my mom, grandma, and aunts would spend hours preparing the most delicious home-cooked, elaborate dishes. These meals shaped the love and gratitude I have for food today.

You may think I was born with these muscles, but I was a skinny and weak kid growing up. I dreamed of having a gorgeous, sculpted body and being strong, powerful, and healthy. I was always interested in nutrition; by the time I was 20, I started reading books and magazines, reviewing the latest research on healthy foods, and taking nutrition courses online. I began lifting weights sporadically at University, but I didn't start my fitness journey until 2007. I was 29 years old, and I had traveled internationally to pursue my love for globetrotting, warm weather, and discoveries. I lived in Bermuda, working full-time as a dental hygienist, where my health and fitness journey began.

On a quest to get in the best shape of my life, I decided to take on a personal fitness challenge and signed up for my first fitness competition. I went all in (as I do with everything in my life) and hired a team of experts, including a trainer, nutritionist, posing coach, costume designer, and fitness choreographer. I had no idea what I was in for, but I had this 5-star pit crew and was super excited to find out—bring on the diet, abs, and spray tan!

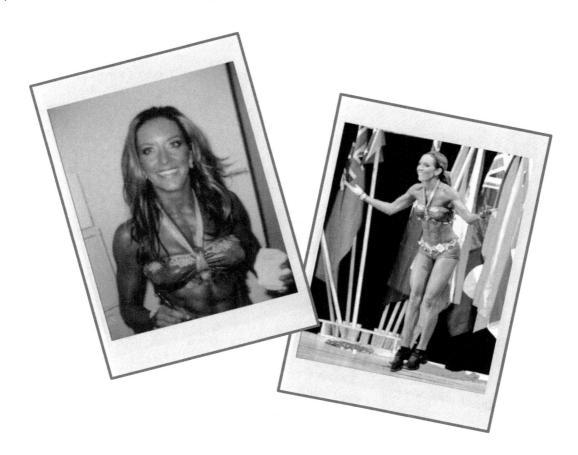

My days for the following eight months were filled to the brim: eat, work, train, cook, sleep, and repeat. I was working full-time as a dental hygienist and exercising between patients—there was a treadmill at the dental office where I worked so I could get my cardio done during my lunch break. Food preparation took hours as I ate up to seven meals per day; I meticulously weighed everything with a food scale. The demands were incredibly grueling. By the time show day arrived, I was 3% body fat and had hunger pains all day. I was taking medication to sleep, I had amenorrhea (I hadn't had a menstrual cycle for six months), and I was desperately craving every kind of unhealthy food you can imagine. I felt exhausted—but I was grinning from ear to ear. I thought, this is how it must feel to be 'fit and strong'; having no appreciation for how much I had compromised my health to achieve the desired look. I was on a high. The competition was a unique, amazing, and new experience! All the hard work and sacrifice paid off when I earned my professional athlete status with the IFBB (International Federation of Bodybuilding). A fire lit inside me—for the first time in my life, I felt passion from the top of my head to the tip of my baby toe! I discovered what moved me. Fitness wasn't just a way to foster the growth of my muscles but a way to promote the development of my mind. As I built my body, I also created a new level of confidence, self-esteem, and a winning, unshakable mentality. Through this experience, I cultivated the ability to establish a 'limitless mindset'—and I knew I would be able to help others do the same. I became hooked on the process of self-improvement and being able to inspire others to better themselves along the way. I started to study nutrition and training and left my career as a dental hygienist to pursue my passion and share my newfound gift with the world. I started my own business as a wellness professional and never looked back.

Now, as exciting as this sounds, there was a dark side to all of this. On the outside, it was all 'glitz and glam,' but it wasn't what it seemed. Behind the scenes, I was struggling to find control of my food. The over-restriction of calories over the last year caught up with me, which is prevalent in the fitness industry as many people, like I unknowingly did, sacrifice their health for an outer physical appearance. My extreme dieting and over-training over those eight months, under the supervision of a team of professionals, had slowly created an unhealthy relationship with food. I treated food as a reward system and believed less was more. I was restricting food and over-exercising in the name of 'health.' After the competitions ended that first year, I couldn't regain control no matter what I did. I just couldn't stop eating. My hormones were severely imbalanced, and I had developed a dirty romance with sugar having extreme cravings at all hours of the day and night. I would eat until I was physically sick, then punish myself with 3 hours of training, and then the next day, I would do it all again. It was a vicious cycle that created a 40-pound weight gain in 3 months; my shredded little body had inflated like a balloon. I was in a food and exercise prison, sprinkling daily self-punishment on myself, and had officially developed a binge eating disorder. I was traumatized and embarrassed. I couldn't understand how this had happened to me. I was educated and grew up in a healthy family without food issues. Little did I know that I had created it entirely, under the supervision of all of those expert professionals, through severe malnourishment and abuse to my body.

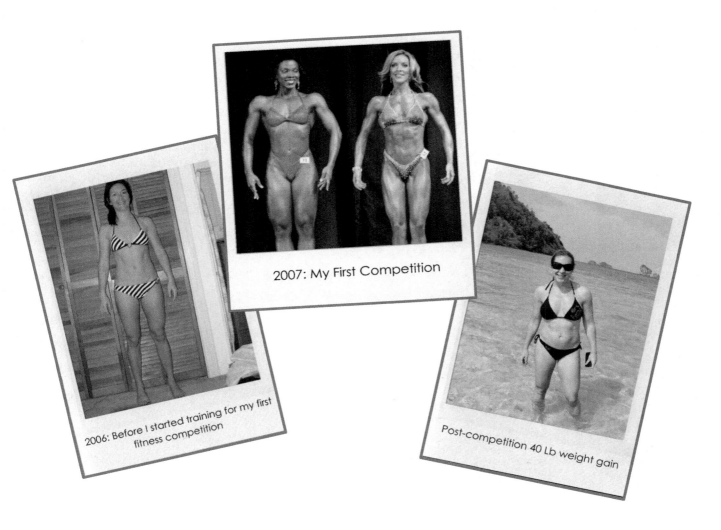

2007: My First Competition

2006: Before I started training for my first fitness competition

Post-competition 40 Lb weight gain

My food philosophy is centered around eating colorful, nutritious foods that taste and make me feel good. How you eat is how you live; how you live is how you eat.

I don't count calories or macros. I prioritize whole foods and limit processed foods as well as those high in saturated fat and sugar. I eat mindfully and consciously with a flexible focus. I also eat as much variety as possible. I crave less, feel better, and have improved my gut health. When creating a meal, I'm always thinking about increasing the meal's nutritional value as much as possible while enhancing flavor without adding excess calories. Our body makes things that it needs from proteins, fats and carbohydrates…not calories. Yet, we put all of our efforts into controlling the 'calories' and meanwhile your body is starving for the one thing no one has taught you how to do - eat for your health. Sure, what I serve up in my kitchen could be scaled back even further to include fewer calories, less fat, and a whole lot less of a lot—but on my journey, I've learned that less is not more when talking about food. To have a lean, healthy body, you don't have to choose a low-calorie meal devoid of nutrition and flavor, leaving you hungry and unsatisfied. A delicious and satisfying 'nutritious' meal that is calorie-focused for your goals will help you achieve your fitness, physique, and health goals while improving your health instead of sacrificing it. Healthy and nutritious food can and should be delicious. Food should taste good and make you feel good— while eating and after. I eat with a focus on nutrient-density, calorie-wise vs. low calorie, simple sugar and gluten-free foods that are highly satisfying, support brain, hormone health, and aging well so I can thrive every day.

I love what I eat, and I eat to live a long, healthy, active life and optimize my well-being. I eat to be a positive role model for my daughter. Food is about bonding with family and friends, enriching my soul, and a connection to myself and the earth through balance and moderation. As you can see, food is a massive part of the intrinsic philosophy weaved through all I do and drives me every day, which is the simple question of 'how can I care for myself at the highest level and become a better version of myself every day.'

Food is a fundamental and exciting part of life. Yes, it's fuel, but it's much more. How we nourish ourselves is the ultimate form of self-respect. Health is a lifestyle, and any beneficial changes we make to how we eat must be sustainable; it's the most powerful tool we have when taking control of our physique and, more importantly, our health. It's information that transforms your biology with every bite, which can activate your potential to heal and thrive or create imbalances that cause health issues and disease. Food is medicine that can balance hormones, reduce inflammation, improve gut health, enhance brain function, and even optimize gene expression. Your amazing body performs all of this awesomeness with no conscious thought on your part! Now that's pretty incredible.

So, if we know this, why are most people constantly yo-yoing on and off diets? A recent study showed that nearly 60 percent of American women tried to lose weight by dieting in the last twelve months (almost 20 percent higher than men).

We also all know that diets don't work! Studies consistently show that 95 percent of individuals who go on a diet end up regaining the weight they lost (and then some). Dieting and unrealistic food intakes, whether a lack of calories or taste, will not lead to a lifestyle that can be maintained for long, at least not happily.

You may ask yourself how and what I eat if I'm not on a 'diet.' The word 'diet' has been ingrained into us from a young age. I started my first diet at University before I was 21! Many cultures condition us to believe that diets are a good thing, and if you're not on a diet, you should be! Crazy right? This mindset is at the root of our relationship with food, and it's time to re-wire that thinking.

With so many fad diets, new eating styles, and science being all over the place, it's overwhelming to know how to eat. Vegan, keto, paleo, Atkins, detox diets, raw food diets, cabbage soup diet, intermittent fasting, hard-core macro counting, low-carb, high-carb, high-fat—ahhh no wonder so many of us are confused about what and how to eat!

I'm here to demystify all this and make eating simple, powerful, and fun. I want you to figure out how to best eat for yourself. In the pages of this book, you'll find so much more than my recipes—you'll learn my nutrition tips, personal strategies, and some common sense that has changed my and my clients' lives. I want you to say goodbye to diets forever and feel empowered and confident, as myself and my clients do, by choosing a dietary lifestyle and developing the food philosophy that serves you, your lifestyle, your health, and your goals.

Before you can truly experience this, it's essential to consider what food means to you.

'You are what you eat' is the old cliché with which you are no doubt familiar, but have you ever realized how profound this notion is and applied it in your life? As a culture, we tend to generally accept that some foods are 'healthy' and some are 'not healthy' (good or bad, as we have incorrectly labeled them), but beyond this level of understanding, there is no deeper meaning behind the way we eat. We eat habitually and not intentionally. We eat without consciously thinking about what this food is doing to our bodies. Many people use apps and fitness trackers that pump out cookie-cutter calories and macros to hit daily. All because we have become disconnected from ourselves , the natural world, and where our food comes from.

Eating with a purpose shouldn't be torturous; it should be rewarding, enjoyable, and sustainable. The good news is that sound science backs these commonsense principles and most experts agree (believe it or not!).

My journey in healing my relationship with food, using it as fuel to achieve extraordinary physical feats, and then experiencing pregnancy has helped me create a profound connection with food on a spiritual level. I've realized that we've somehow come to a point in the human experience where we no longer intuitively know what is correct for us to eat.

Let that sink in for a moment.

Why are we the only species on Earth to have this problem? No single animal living in their natural environment is overweight or suffering a chronic illness due to their diet. They know exactly what to eat. They're in touch with the innate intelligence that drives their food choices, and as a result, they thrive. Of course, a tiger in the Serengeti doesn't have access to toxic convenience food or the McDonald's drive-thru, but you get my point. If this alone doesn't show how spiritually disconnected we have become, then I don't know what will.

Food is very personal and has come to mean different things to all of us. How we choose to eat or not eat reflects our ethical and religious principles and the amount of respect we have for ourselves, the environment, and others. For myself and my clients, pondering our eating habits in a meaningful manner has created insight into a deeper understanding of who we are.

Food is also profoundly political and is at the center of several funding questions for political philosophy. Here are some things to consider. The challenges that food consumption poses to the environment. For example, did you know that factory farming is responsible for a higher rate of pollution than airfare travel? Food production, distribution, and retail contribute to some of the poorest working conditions for workers worldwide. Federal food policies in the

US, and many other countries, encourage Big Food (the brands that dominate the production and sale of packaged food and drink) and put private profit over public health. The food system is the most significant global industry generating over $18 trillion annually. So yes, your food purchases matter.

These thoughts have created my food philosophy, and I challenge you to ask yourself what food means to you. Loving what you eat at every meal should meet your body's needs (without excess) and those of your mind, heart, and soul. Why would you eat the same tomorrow if you don't love what you ate today?

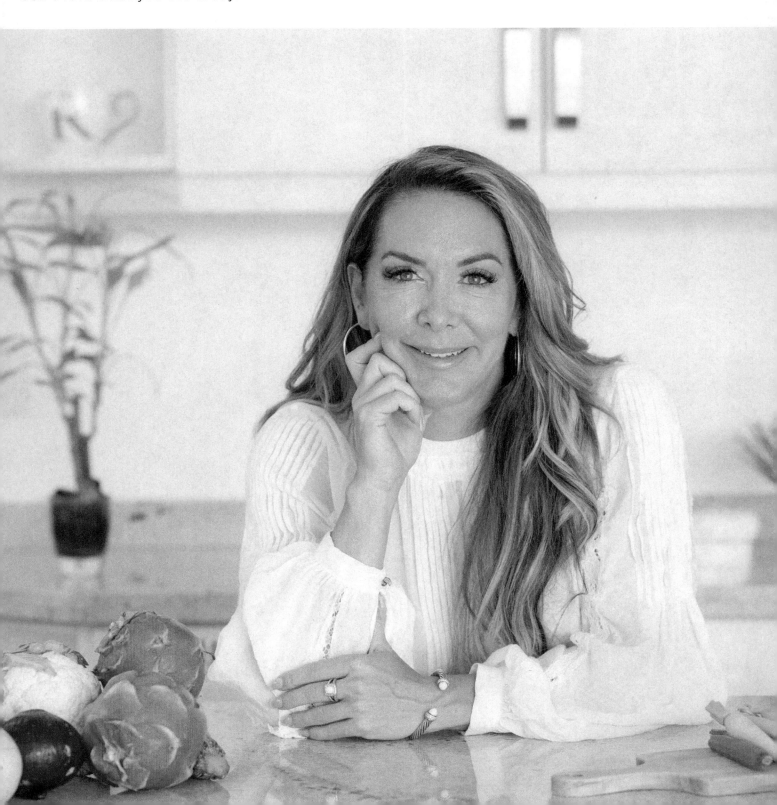

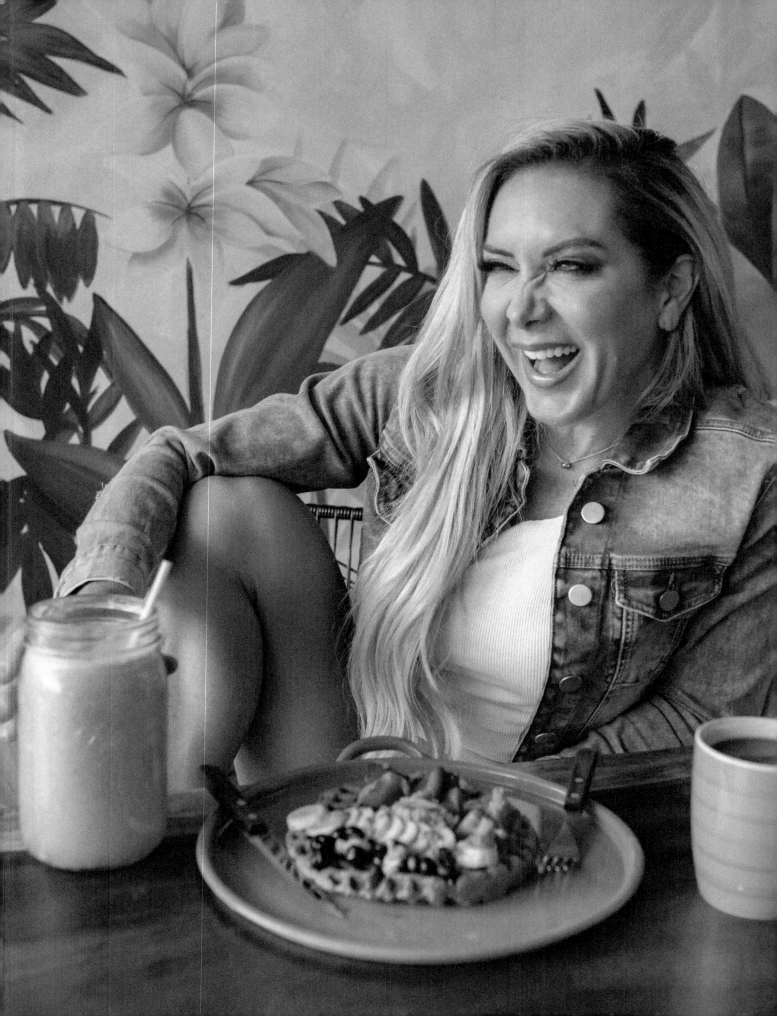

HOW TO EAT TO THRIVE

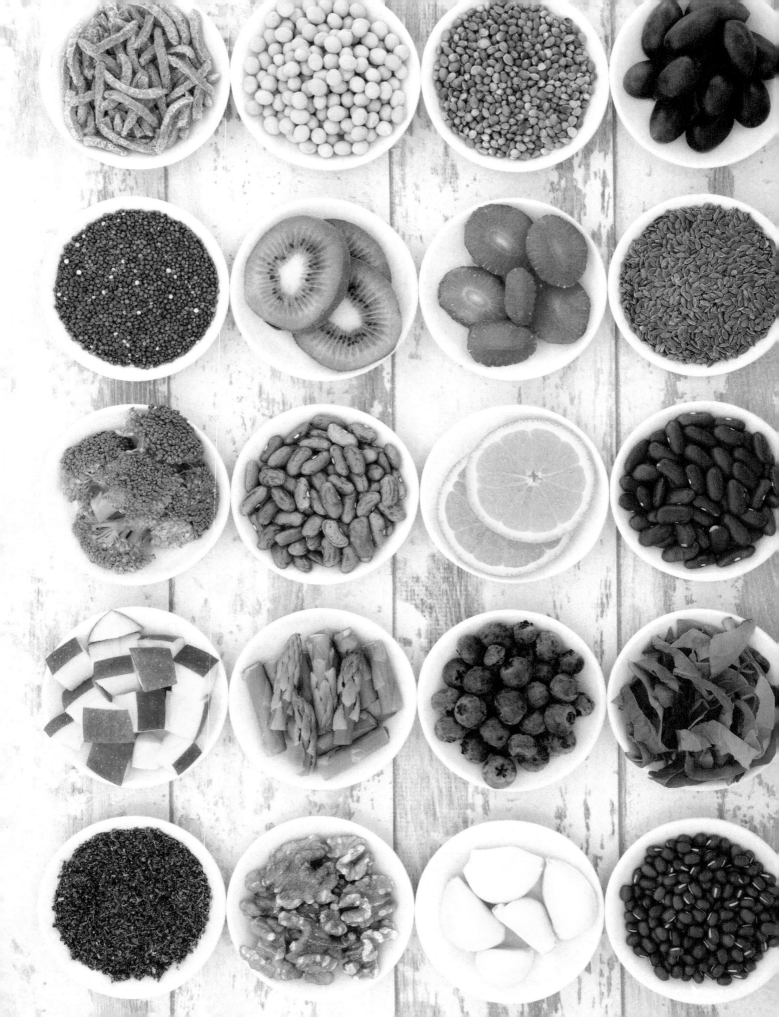

Macronutrients, Micronutrients, and Calculating your Energy Requirements

It's important to have a basic understanding of these nutrition principles to learn how to eat. I'm going to keep it as simple and exciting as possible!

Every single food has macronutrients and micronutrients. Eating a beautiful balance of both is one of the key elements to achieving optimal health and thriving every day.

What are Macros?

We all require energy to function, and as you can guess, that energy comes from the foods we eat. Macronutrients are the nutrients that your body requires in large amounts and are the main elements of nutrition.

There are three macronutrients. Each has different properties and functions. They contain essential vitamins, minerals, and of course, energy.

> **Proteins** = 4 Calories / gram
> **Carbohydrates** = 4 Calories / gram
> **Fats** = 9 Calories / gram

Macronutrients break down into smaller forms during digestion; protein into amino acids, carbs into glucose, and fats into fatty acids and glycerol. They're then ready for absorption through the small intestine.

It's important to mention fiber and alcohol, which aren't officially considered macronutrients, but they do yield energy:

> **Fiber** = 2 Calories/ gram
> **Alcohol** = 7 Calories / gram

Fiber, or bulk roughage, is a type of carbohydrate found naturally in plant foods and isn't digestible. However, bacteria in the large intestine ferment some of this, leading to a minor energy release. Its importance shouldn't be underestimated as it's very important for optimal health. Fiber comes in two forms, soluble and insoluble. Soluble fiber absorbs water and causes digestion to slow down while insoluble fiber—you guessed it—repels water and provides bulk to your stool.

Alcohol generally contains no vitamins or minerals but still contributes to energy due to ethanol.

Track your Energy Balance

It's valuable to calculate your BMR (basal metabolic rate) and TDEE (total daily energy expenditure) to estimate how many calories you burn based on your physical activity level. Think of it as doing an energy audit. Knowing your approximate BMR and caloric output every day is important in understanding your general caloric requirements.

To calculate this go to https://tdeecalculator.net (I find this to be the most accurate calculator online) and enter your height, weight, and an estimate of your physical activity level. Be honest with your activity levels without under or overestimating them to get the most accurate result. The calculator is going to give you an estimated maintenance calorie number. It's important to remember that these values are always an estimate and the only way to determine your true resting metabolic rate is with Metabolic Testing. It's also important to note that foods are influenced by how they're grown and prepared, and every person has a different calorie-burning potential determined by their age, weight, muscle mass, health status, and many other factors. There is no way to be 100% accurate when calculating Calories in versus Calories out. Furthermore, this shouldn't be your ultimate goal, or it will become obsessive. However, tracking your energy balance over a short period is a valuable and effective way to learn how many calories your body needs.

Improving your Metabolic Health

Metabolism is the process that your body uses to transform food to energy your body uses to function. Our metabolic rates are individual and unique. They also fluctuate throughout our lives. A slow metabolic rate is a real thing that can come from chronic dieting, disordered eating patterns, unbalanced macro and micronutrients, certain medication, inactivity, low muscle mass and poor thyroid health. If you feel your metabolism is slower than it should be, don't stress. Unless you have been diagnosed with a thyroid disorder, it's often not as complicated to restore your metabolism and vitality as you may think. The first step is understanding the basics with energy balance above and then making simple, but profound lifestyle changes that support the upregulation of your metabolism.

After nearly two decades in the wellness space I will tell you that this comes down to optimal self care - wholesome food (like the meals found in the pages of this book), proper hydration, appropriate exercise, stress management, balanced lifestyle and sufficient sleep. The greatest parameter contributing to your success is consistency. So don't overthink this or think you're doomed if your metabolism is slow and just get started making small changes to living a healthier lifestyle.

If you think you may have a thyroid disorder and have never checked your thyroid function with a blood test I suggest having this tested as the main job of the thyroid is to control your metabolism. The thyroid creates the hormones T4 and T3 to control your metabolism and these hormones work throughout the body to tell the body's cells how much energy to use. So as you can imagine, it's pretty important that your thyroid health is optimal. This is one of the blood tests I request for baseline information prior to working with a client. I've had very favorable outcomes with my own body as well as my clients with appropriate lifestyle and nutrition changes over time. To learn more about the types of foods that support thyroid health head to page 100.

One of the many beauties of our bodies is they are incredibly good at adapting to meet the demands placed on them. Our bodies are always working for us (or wanting to work for us!), not against us. If you need to repeat that sentence do so, as it may just serve as a reminder of how amazing your body is.

When Monday comes around, it's great to be prepared with healthy food for your week. I love the expression 'If you fail to plan, you plan to fail!' Meal planning can seem daunting, but the good news is it doesn't have to be! Sitting down to plan your meals and menu (with all these delicious recipes!) for the entire week instead of at the moment for each meal will help you save time and money and is key to achieving success with your health goals. I plan my meals every week, without fail—it's now a weekly ritual we have that happens without thinking (yay for healthy habit creation!). And other than fruits and vegetables for snacking and the occasional bottle of wine, I won't digress from what's on my grocery list. I use whole, unprocessed foods and always try to shop for local and organic products. I often pre-order organic local produce online to save time and money and to support my local farmers; which helps me stay focused and organized. I tend to eat in-season and fresh. In Cancun, at the time of publishing, we spend about $125USD per week on groceries for the 3 of us. That excludes our meals in restaurants which we do 2-4 times per week.

These are my four steps to simple and successful meal planning:

1. First, plan your meals, select your recipes, and record them in your weekly meal planner. Dinners can become leftovers for lunch the next day; this is where you get clear on how your meals will look for the week.
2. Make your grocery list. I love making lists. This way, I don't forget anything I need. Lists also allow you to group items together, so you're not wasting time at the store going back and forth between aisles and departments. Save time and get my Grocery List which has every ingredient from all of the recipes organized in a pre-made list. HERE
3. Next, shop for fresh ingredients and any pantry staples you need to stock up on.
4. Lastly, prepare your meals.

My Step-by-Step Menu Planning Method:

I typically take advantage of the weekend to master my three-step approach to meal planning:

Plan on Friday: Firstly, Look at the week ahead, roughly assess your schedule and the nights you plan to cook at home and the nights you plan to go out, what days you'll have leftovers (oh yeah, I'm a huge fan of leftovers—the gift that keeps on giving!), and then decide on the recipes you want to make. I recommend planning a variety of both warm, cooked foods and cold, raw foods for optimal gut health and nutrient absorption. Write them into your weekly meal planner. Marcelo and I sit down with our menu planner and enjoy this time together planning our meals for the week. We also chose the meals we plan to have in restaurants, which are the busy days when we prefer not to cook. We have eight different weekly menu planners pre-made and tend to rotate them with slight adjustments. As a meal planning devotee, I can tell you that this is the first step in feeling empowered, organized, and totally in charge of mealtime for the week ahead. When getting started, I recommend trying one to two new recipes that look exciting from my book every week. Then, once you've mastered them, start adding a new recipe every week. These recipes will become the tools in your toolkit. The more you make them, the more confident you will become and the easier preparation becomes. Soon you'll be cooking like us—without even using the recipes anymore! #MealBoss Get a meal plan for your goals with the recipes in the book here https://ryallgraber.com/shop.

Shop on Saturday: After you have a chance to plan your recipes, check the pantry and make a grocery list, then head to the grocery store to shop or order online. This trip to the store is going to set you up for success for the week ahead. The beauty of shopping on Saturday is that it eliminates several after-work trips to the store during the week. Maybe you'll need to stop by the market later in the week to pick up some fresh items, but the Saturday shop tackles the bulk of the week's groceries. Ordering online is a great hack to save time for those few mid-week items! Since afternoons tend to mean more shoppers and longer lines, I like to go first thing in the morning or on Saturday night. And don't shop hungry—you may end up with some impulse, unhealthy items that weren't on your list!

Prep on Sunday: A quick Sunday 'prep session' in the kitchen helps put your plan into action and makes weeknight cooking feel a lot easier. This can be as simple as cutting up the veggies for a stir-fry, pre-making your protein pizza base, baking one of my sweet potato recipes, tossing some marinated protein in your air fryer, or cooking one of my soups or chilies, so all you have to do is reheat it on Tuesday night. If you work out of the home and run on a hectic schedule, cooking fresh meals daily may not be an option for you—and that's ok! I suggest you cook larger quantities or a variety of foods to use in different ways throughout the week. Then, create your lunches and dinners. You can either just pop them in the fridge or the freezer. You can pre-portion your prepped meals to ensure your portion sizes are appropriate and even freeze some things in bulk, which can work well if you have a family as well. Some of my favorite frozen items are Fish Bites (substitute chicken or turkey), Blueberry Maple Turkey Breakfast Patties, Egg Bites, and Sweet Potato Fries. All that's left to do then is heat them. I always start my day with one of my fresh, nourishing breakfast recipes. I do some bulk preparation of vegetables for salad contents on Sunday and Wednesday (depending on what our menu looks like for the week), and we prepare most dinners fresh with recipes. If I'm having a super busy week, I may also do some bulk prep of carbs (my favorites are in the sides section!). These are portable nutrition options like my Superfood Cookies, Breakfast Brownies, and Overnight Oats, or one of my protein muffin recipes that make a perfect, on-the-go snack paired with a piece of fruit and I'll also prepare some basic chicken and fish with my home-made Herb Marinades for flavor. We also precook certain staples like tomato sauce and salsa and top up any fresh dressings, dips, and marinades to save time.

This is my system - it may work for you, and it may not. Think of this as a framework versus 'rules' and use it to get started with and then adjust and refine your system as you go to make it fit your lifestyle.

The Benefits of Planning Your Meals

Tackling meal planning saves you time during the week, and ultimately it will be a lot easier to stay on track with healthy eating. When you've got your menu and a meal preparation plan, you know what you're eating, and it takes the thinking and planning out of it. If I've prepared my meals, it allows me to feel relaxed, and I achieve my goals a lot faster. There's nothing worse than 'hanger' setting in and not having a meal ready. Food prep has taught me so much about nutrition and cooking! Knowing there's a healthy, balanced, nutritious meal waiting for me helps me avoid mindless snacking in between meals. It also helps with portion control and has helped me to minimize binging-type behaviors. Nourishing your body with delicious and nutritious meals is the ultimate form of self-respect. Making what you put in your body a priority is a rewarding part of your self-care and fitness journey—so enjoy it.

You Did It! Now Do it Again!

Meal planning isn't complex, but it's not a walk in the park either—especially when you're new to it. As with anything in which we want to succeed, it takes our investment of time. But when your health is a priority, this should feel non-negotiable. You may feel a bit nervous, but you should also feel excited! If you purchased this book to make your life in the kitchen a bit calmer, you're already well on your way. Every time you go through the meal planning process, you learn what not to do, where to improve next week, what you can skip, how to save time, and how to customize the entire practice to fit your family's needs. It's a process, and you learn as you go. Like anything, practice makes perfect, and continuing to do it only helps you improve.

How to Shop Like a Pro

Grocery shopping is one of life's never-ending chores, but it can make all the difference when living a healthy life. When it's done effectively you'll be surprised how simple (and how fun it can be!). This section is full of my tips and strategies to help you up your grocery shopping game.

My Tips to Shop Like A Pro

1. Make a List. As you've learned above, one of the most important parts of any healthy meal planning routine is creating the grocery list and going grocery shopping. If you're new to eating healthy or trying to get more organized in the kitchen, perfecting your grocery list is easily one of the most practical ways you can change your eating habits and is imperative for a successful shop. You've got to stay on track and avoid impulse purchases in those junk aisles! Get my Grocery List Here https://ryallgraber.com/shop.

2. Choose Quality Foods. How and where your food was grown has a massive impact on the nutrients it will provide to your body. Words like 'natural' or 'free range' don't tell you much. See the section on third-party labels and certifications for more on this.

3. Eating on a budget. Eating healthy on a budget can be a challenge, especially when buying higher-quality products. However, you can certainly eat healthfully and follow a budget. It's possible to even save money and eat healthier, especially if you've been purchasing a lot of convenience foods or eating out frequently. You're now eating whole foods so they cost less. To save money, make your own salad dressings (see page 312), buy in bulk, shop at local farmers' markets, buy a fruit and veggie wash to remove pesticides (if you can't buy organic), and stick to your list. A recent study showed that online grocery shopping saved an average of 15% more than shopping in the store because we spend less if we aren't browsing. This makes sense as it's easier to see sales and compare shops—not to mention saving the fuel cost, time, and no traffic!

4. Stick to the outside aisles for the most nutrient-dense foods—it really does work!

5. Learn how to properly read your food labels. Don't rely on health claims stated on labels and fancy marketing as your guide. Instead, learn a few simple label-reading tips to choose healthy minimally processed foods and drinks.

How to Read the Nutrition Facts Label

Food labels on pre-packaged foods can seem perplexing, misleading, and difficult to decipher. Whether you are looking to limit your sugar, improve your health, heal your gut, reduce calories, or increase your fiber intake, it's imperative that you can make sense of the numbers, ingredients, and nutritional information packed into that tiny box. If you're serious about your health, you'll want to get serious about reading your labels.

In the US, the Food and Drug Administration (FDA) requires a Nutrition Facts label on most packaged foods and beverages. Knowing how to read the Nutrition Facts panel comes down to quantity and quality—'How much?' and 'Of what?' At the top of the Nutrition Facts label, you will find the total number of servings in the container and the food or beverage serving size.

WHAT'S LISTED?

- **Serving size:** The amount of the product typically consumed at once.
- **Calories:** The number of calories, or energy, provided by a single serving. 2,000 calories are the average daily reference amount, based on the caloric intake recommended for many average Americans. This is not a recommendation of how much to eat as this is unique to your body, eating style, and goals.
- **Percent Daily Value:** The Daily Value is how much of a given nutrient you should either aim to reach (for example, dietary fiber) or keep below (like sodium). Knowing how much of that amount is in a given food can help you keep track.
- **Nutrients:** Fats, carbohydrates, protein, and cholesterol, as well as select vitamins and minerals.

A

Nutrition Facts

8 servings per container
Serving size   2/3 cup (55g)

Amount per serving
Calories   230

	% Daily Value*
Total Fat 8g	**10%**
Saturated Fat 1g	**5%**
Trans Fat 0g	
Cholesterol 0mg	**0%**
Sodium 160g	**7%**
Total Carbohydrate 37g	**13%**
Dietary Fiber 4g	**14%**
Total Sugars 12g	
Includes 10g Added Sugars	**20%**
Protein 3g	
Vitamin D 2mcg	10%
Calcium 260mg	20%
Iron 8mg	45%
Potassium 240mg	6%

*The % Daily Value (DV) tells you how much a nutrient in a serving of food contributes to a daily diet. 2,000 calories a day is used for general nutrition advice.

B

Nutrition Facts

2 servings per container
Serving size   1 cup (255g)

Calories	Per serving **220**		Per container **440**	
		% DV*		% DV*
Total Fat	5g	**6%**	10g	**13%**
Saturated Fat	2g	**10%**	4g	**20%**
Trans Fat	0g		0g	
Cholesterol	15mg	**5%**	30mg	**10%**
Sodium	240mg	**10%**	480mg	**21%**
Total Carb.	35g	**13%**	70g	**25%**
Dietary Fiber	6g	**21%**	12g	**43%**
Total Sugars	7g		14g	
Incl. Added Sugars	4g	**8%**	8g	**16%**
Protein	9g		18g	
Vitamin D	5mcg	25%	10mcg	50%
Calcium	200mg	15%	400mg	30%
Iron	1mg	6%	2mg	10%
Potassium	470mg	10%	940mg	20%

* The % Daily Value (DV) tells you how much a nutrient in a serving of food contributes to a daily diet. 2,000 calories a day is used for general nutrition advice.

The remainder of the label information is usually based on one serving of the food or beverage (see Food Label A). However, if the container has more than one serving but typically might be consumed in one sitting—such as a pint of ice cream—the label will have two additional columns (see Food Label B). The first of these columns lists the calories and nutrients in one

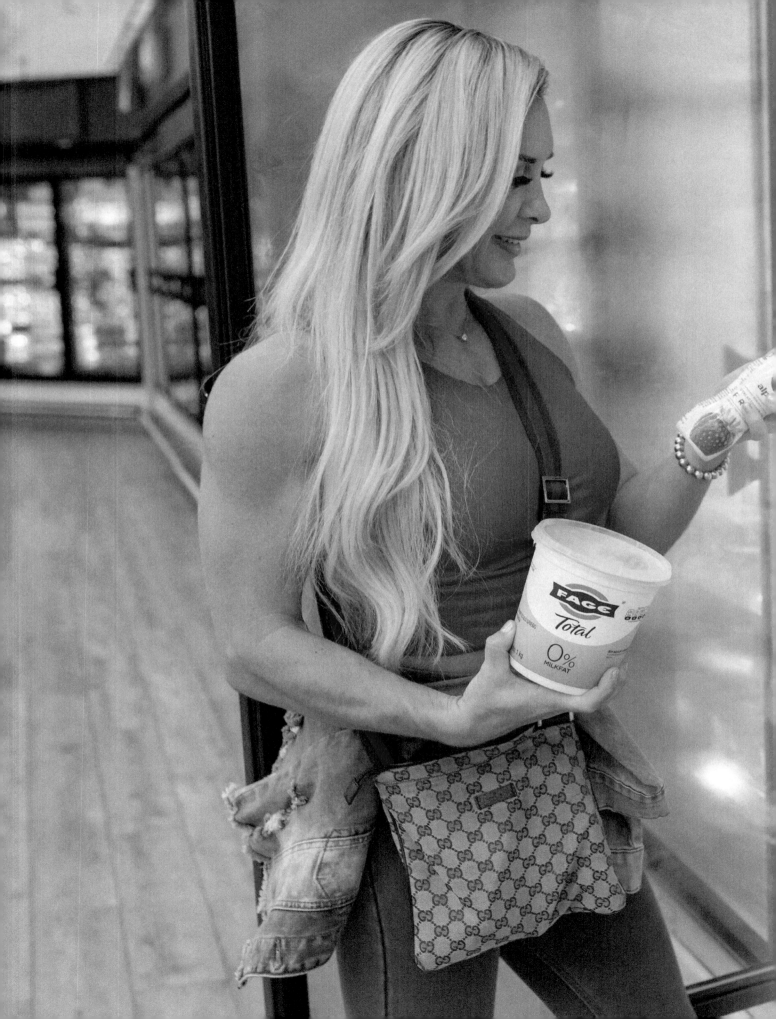

serving. The second lists the same information for the entire container. If you eat a whole package of food that contains two servings, you will get twice as many calories, nutrients, sugar, and fat as in one serving.

When I make a quick scan of a label, I'm looking at the following things:

- **Total and Added Sugar:** Aim for as low as possible, from a natural source, and avoid added sugar. Added sugars are a big issue in our food supply right now—it's literally in everything hence why diabetes has become an epidemic. This is one of the most important things to check. In the US, by law, the label marks the difference between total sugar and added sugar; however, food manufacturers in many other countries (like Canada) are not required to include the amount of added sugar a product contains. This is where added sugars are included in all kinds of products (even bread and yogurt!) for added taste. One teaspoon is 4 grams of sugar and many yogurts on the market today have a whopping 17-20 grams of total sugar per serving.
- **Dietary Fiber:** As high as possible. Most people are not getting near enough. I aim for 28 g daily and love products that have a lot of fiber to help with happy bowel movements, feelings of fullness, and to reduce total carbs. To calculate net carbs, you want to subtract the fiber from the total carbs as it's not digestible. When you can find a calorie-smart, high protein, and high fiber food you're winning! One of my favorites is lentil pasta.
- **Calories:** Reasonable calories per portion. I don't look for low-calorie packaged foods, but instead for calorie-wise foods. For example, if 100 g serving is 700 calories I wouldn't pick it.
- **Saturated Fat:** Less than 10 g and, ideally, as low as possible with healthier fats like unsaturated fats.
- **Trans Fat:** None. Avoid this completely. The good news is that by 2023, the World Health Organization has called for the elimination of all artificial sources of trans fats from food products worldwide.
- **Sodium:** As low as possible. I reference the daily value advised by Harvard T.H. Chan School of Public Health, which is 1500 mg. You'll add sodium to your whole food meals so you don't want to be consuming much more than this.
- **Macronutrients:** I am more likely to purchase food that has higher protein. I'll take a closer look at the ingredient list to determine the fat and carbohydrate quality of a product.

No label? No problem. You want 90% of your food items from whole food sources and let that last 10% come from minimally processed foods. Some of my favorites that I couldn't live without are sugar-free ketchup and syrup, rice cakes, avocado oil-based mayo, dark chocolate, and nitrate-free pre-sliced turkey breast. You can find nutrition information for fresh fruits and vegetables on the USDA website (https://www.usda.gov/topics/food-and-nutrition).

How to Read the Ingredient List

The ingredients in packaged food and beverage items are listed separately from (and often below) the Nutrition Facts label. This information lists each ingredient in the product by its common or usual name, and in descending order by weight. That is, the ingredient that weighs the most is listed first, and the ingredient that weighs the least is listed last.

Unfortunately, there are still additives in our foods that are harmful to our health. Lawmakers, however, claim that not enough scientific evidence has been collected over a sufficiently long period to give reason to ban these substances. This is slowly changing but, in the meantime, it's imperative we educate ourselves so we can make informed choices instead of being victimized by the food industry. This is the only way in which we can protect ourselves and our loved ones. This is how we influence the direction of the conventional food industry and the range

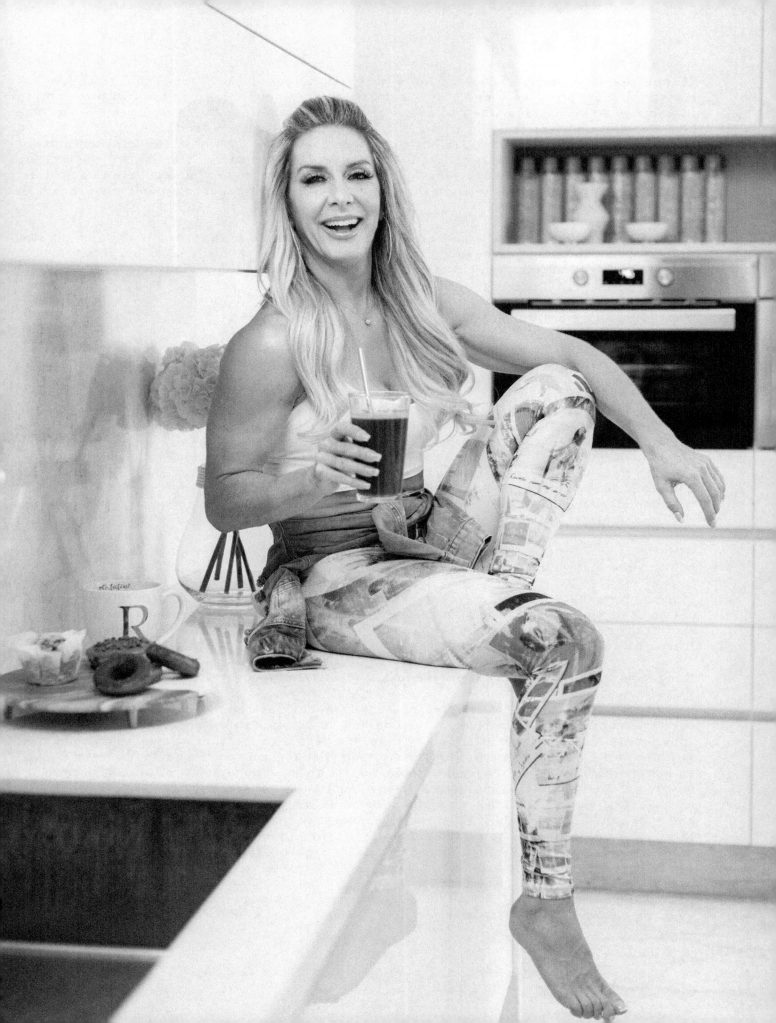

Changing your behaviors and thoughts takes time, and it also takes practice. It's not something most of us learn and practice growing up. Although we're all born with the ability to know when to eat and when to stop eating—and know what is satisfying—we've become disconnected and less trusting of our intuition with diet culture, social media, family, and friends. 'Clean your plate or you're not getting dessert' is a conditioned thought that most of us have after being told this as children. This is where the disconnect started. But the exciting thing is that we can change any behavior or thoughts that aren't serving us. With dedication, consistency and a deep desire to change we can rewire our thoughts around any process to create a desirable outcome.

You're going to fail. But you're also going to learn. Failures are always the best opportunities to learn. Be compassionate and kind to yourself along the way. Get prepared to get uncomfortable when you let go of the structure and start trusting yourself more. You can and will do this.

What is Intuitive Eating?

According to the National Eating Disorders Association, intuitive eating is about trusting your body to make food choices that feel good for you, without judging yourself or being influenced by diet culture.

Intuitive eating is a simple idea. It means that you make peace and are comfortable with all types of food. Unlike traditional 'diets' that restrict certain foods, intuitive eating requires you to stop looking at food as good or bad. You instead learn to see food as healthy and unhealthy while finding a healthy balance by listening to your body and eating what feels right for you. Now, this doesn't mean you just eat whatever you want, anytime you want! If your body is asking for pizza and donuts all day, it's time to push the reset button. Start to replace these foods slowly with the yummy goodness you'll see in the recipe section and keep the occasional pizza and donut as a part of your nutrition (if you love them!). Then you'll transition into more healthy and wholesome eating and less anxiety and distress. The idea with intuitive eating is that you're focused on foods that support your physical and mental health as well as your goals.

Studies show that cultivating a daily practice of mindfulness can help reduce stress, binge eating, and emotional eating. I'm telling you; this is powerful. Learning this skill is your Mac-daddy tool when it comes to finding freedom from food prison and truly being able to eat from a place of empowerment.

Hunger and Satiety Cues, Food Awareness, and Satisfaction

You can't run a Ferrari on empty. Your body needs fuel and frequency is going to be determined by your hunger levels. Learning how to monitor your hunger between meals and your satiety levels during meals is a way to form a deeper connection with your body and start to listen to its needs. If you want to master this, I suggest using two tools—a journal and/or an alarm. Track your hunger levels so you can follow your daily patterns and learn to check in with yourself. Especially if you're that busy boss bee who is so busy that they forget to eat all day! This is going to take time and will be some work, but it's just for the first 7-14 days, and then you'll have established a better connection and this is going to become low-level thinking. Think of this as going to school—it's an investment in learning and then you've got it! We want this to become a habit that you just 'do' naturally versus having to think about it, as you'll have to do in the beginning.

I teach this as a scale system and have my clients rate this on a scale of 1-10. When you feel your hunger is around 7, you want to have a meal. If you're under 7, you'll feel like you're force-feeding. On the contrary, if you leave it too long, it may quickly escalate to a 10 (hangry!). You'll likely find that your portion size isn't satiating. You'll notice an energy dip, overeat, and will want sugar because your blood sugar has dropped a bit too low. Sometimes thirst can be misinterpreted as hunger as well. So, make sure you're hydrating between meals. This is also the time when hunger and fatigue intersect and many people reach for a cuppa java. You immediately feel better, but this isn't going to sustain you for long. Instead, you'll get a huge drop in energy and brain function because you're not giving your body the nutrients it needs. Not to mention the stress that too much caffeine causes on our adrenal glands.

Set an alarm to go off every two hours and check in with yourself. Are you hungry yet? Decide from there if you can wait longer or want to have a meal. Trust your body and permit yourself to eat when it lets you know you're hungry. Hunger is the cue that guides me when I eat all of my meals—starting with the first and last meal of the day. Each day may be different based on exercise, sleep, stress levels, or hormones—and that's ok. Remember there are no rules around feeding times. It's what makes you feel your best.

I use the same scale with satiety during eating. Satiety means your level of fullness. You want to be able to stop eating at a comfortable level of fullness, and you also want to be able to identify if you need to eat more food to feel satiated. To do this, you want to eat slowly and chew slowly. Take time to savor the experience of eating; enjoy all the different tastes and textures. Put away your phone and anything that's distracting you. Stay aware when you're eating to get the most from the experience. In time and with practice you won't feel like overeating.

Food awareness can also be considered on the same spectrum. If we lose awareness, then we disconnect and eat mindlessly. For example, you open up a bag of M&M's™. You want a small portion to sprinkle on your protein pancakes, but then you say, "ah forget it, I've already had 5" and binge on two bags. If we're hyper-aware, say at a level 9/10, then we're food obsessed, leading to either restricting, weighing, and/or tracking everything we eat. For a healthy relationship with food, we want our awareness to sit in the middle around 5. If you want the M&M's™, you're able to have a small portion and stop when you feel satisfied.

Ever find yourself snacking right after dinner? When we're not satisfied, we will either continue to pick at foods or overindulge. This is a different feeling than being hungry. When you feel satisfied and happy, you'll know you've had enough. If you're not feeling satisfied, pause and ask yourself what it is that you're craving. Sometimes it may be carbs (a handful of berries will likely curb it), but most often it will be fat, and something as simple as adding some ghee to your vegetables, whole grain bread (my fav!), Guilt-free Chocolate Pudding made with avocado (get it on page 336), or enjoying a square of dark chocolate, will do the trick. When you start to feel satisfied with every meal, you won't continue to eat. You won't think about food. You'll start to get comfortable with the thought that one square of chocolate won't make you gain fat, just like one salad won't make you lean. If you can find the right balance for yourself, you'll be able to master eating, for life.

Another matter of interest is the fact that progesterone increases the week before a woman's menstrual cycle, this increases metabolism, and hunger can surge. Instead of blaming PMS and eating yourself into a carb coma the week before your period, or ignoring your hunger cues, simply expect to feel a bit hungrier and plan to increase your calories from healthy carbs that week to help curb your hunger. If only I had known this sooner… Every coach I worked with before I self-coached followed the same programs with women and men, without any regard for the differences in our hormones. Being in tune with your body is invaluable!

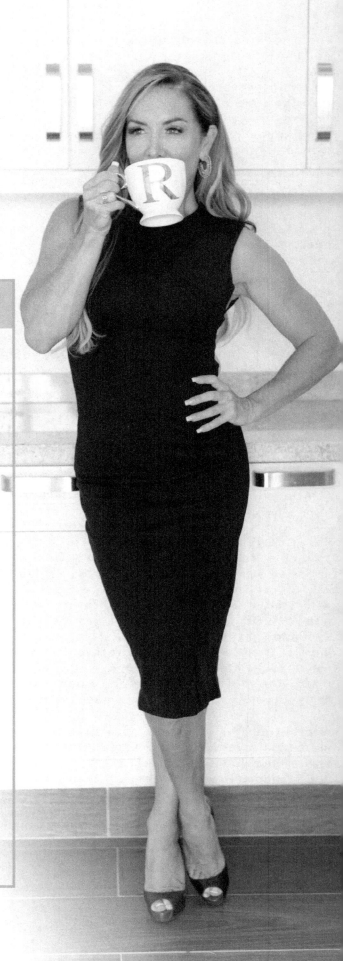

Doing the Inner Work

It's important to do the inner work here and be honest with yourself by reflecting on your behaviors. Some of them might be guiding you down a path you don't want to take. It's common for healthy habits and behaviors to become unhealthy, negatively impact our health and well-being, and conflict with our core values. Maybe you're currently tracking your food and think it's working for you. This is great if you feel happy. However, if you're unsure if you need to strengthen your relationship with food here are some thoughts and behaviors that can help you take a deeper look at your eating patterns.

BEHAVIORS THAT INDICATE YOU NEED TO IMPROVE YOUR RELATIONSHIP WITH FOOD

You spend most of your day thinking about food and your next meal. Your thoughts around food have become obsessive.

Skipping meals to 'cut calories' but then you binge eat, or uncontrollably eat, later that night.

Cutting out all 'bad foods' for too long and then binge eating on sugar.

When you start to eat unhealthy food, you feel like you've 'ruined your day,' so you continue eating unhealthy foods for the rest of the day (all or none mindset).

Restricting unhealthy foods that you enjoy.

Ignoring your hunger cues outside of your mealtimes. You normalize this feeling and the disconnect from it.

Doing extra cardio to punish yourself for eating extra calories the day before.

Weighing every single food you eat and tracking calories. You view food as a calculation to hit vs nourishment.

You've lost your period (amenorrhea) because you aren't eating enough healthy calories to support your activity levels.

You remove yourself from social situations because you're afraid to navigate food outside of your kitchen. This would create anxiety for you.

Put your phone down when eating as this is a distraction, and you want to be more mindful and present while eating.

Sit down when you eat. Eat slowly.

If you love and want the donut, have it. Focus on the smell, taste, and texture. Enjoy it, fully and without guilt.

Stop labeling foods as good or bad. You are not 'good' for eating a salad and 'bad' for eating ice cream. This can lead to a slippery slope of determining your self-worth based on the last bite of food you ate and can get you in the fast lane towards an unhealthy relationship with food quickly. This often leads to people feeling like they align with that moral standing when they eat certain foods. It's not only unhealthy, but also it's ridiculous if you think about it. Foods are simply healthy and unhealthy and a healthy balance of both is the objective.

Put the food scale away if it's becoming an unhealthy obsession for you.

Learn your hunger and satiety cues and eyeball your portion sizes according to your goals. You don't need to know the exact calorie macronutrient breakdown of every food item you eat.

Unfollow social media accounts that post too many body checks as this could be a trigger to restrict food intake again and go back into unhealthy behaviors.

Stop labeling foods as good or bad. You are not 'good' for eating a salad and 'bad' for eating ice cream. This can lead to a slippery slope of determining your self-worth based on the last bite of food you ate and can get you in the fast lane towards an unhealthy relationship with food quickly. This often leads to people feeling like they align with that moral standing when they eat certain foods. It's not only unhealthy, but also it's ridiculous if you think about it. Foods are simply healthy and unhealthy and a healthy balance of both is the objective.

Putting these principles into practice

There's no better place to do this than in a restaurant. With these principles in check, it's possible to go out for a meal and stay on track with your goals. In the same respect, it's also possible to go out and enjoy an unhealthy meal while staying in control and feeling good about it.

If your goal is to keep it healthy, I suggest choosing a restaurant that has a healthy option on the menu that suits your nutrition goals. You can choose what you want to eat before you go out if this makes you feel more confident about not ordering an unhealthy meal spur of the moment. Never go to dinner hungry as it's harder to flex that willpower muscle when you're hangry. Eat a small meal before heading out or have a protein shake to curb your hunger.

Be wary of items that are labeled 'gluten-free' or 'sugar-free.' This classification doesn't necessarily mean it's any healthier. Often you'll ask the server what they've used in place of wheat for a gluten-free item, and they have no idea. Last week I tried a new 'healthy pizza' restaurant that claimed they had a cauliflower pizza crust, only to learn that it also had regular flour incorporated into the crust. I also see 'sugar-free' a lot. When I inquire about the ingredients, they've used natural sugars like agave syrup; which we know aren't sugar-free. Request that your sauces and dressings stay on the side as this will help you control how much you add to your meal. If you want to keep it lighter, swap the fries or potatoes for extra vegetables or a salad to get that extra fiber in!

Non-GMO

At this time there's not enough research about what GMO's (genetically modified organisms) actually do to our health. Personally I chose to avoid GMO's as I don't take chances with my health. A great way to avoid them is to buy organic. The other way is to look for the label which is this non-GMO Project Verified seal of approval. When you see this label you can feel assured you're avoiding genetically altered food, even if it's not organic. If you can't buy organic this is the next best thing.

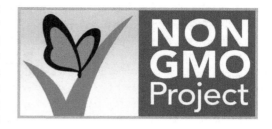

Grass-Fed or Pasture Raised

Grass-Fed refers to beef, goat, bison, lamb, sheep and dairy products while 'pasture-raised' refers to poultry, pork and eggs. These designations mean that the product is from an animal that was raised eating its natural diet outdoors. This is the type of animal protein you ideally want to be consuming. When a cow is exclusively being fed corn (when they're meant to eat grass) their bodies become inflamed and unhappy and this is the quality of the meat we consume. When shopping, look for grass-fed meat and pasture-raised poultry.

Wild-Caught and Sustainably Harvested Seafood

The health benefits of wild-caught seafood are endless. Wild-caught fish have greater nutritional value than farmed. Farmed fish are fed corn and soy which creates higher levels of inflammatory omega 6 fatty acids that are passed on to you. They also have nearly undetectable amounts of omega-3 fatty acids and contain high levels of contaminants. I always recommend wild-caught seafood, but if farmed fish is your only option, then look for those raised without antibiotics and hormones. Wild-caught salmon, anchovies, mackerel, sardines and herring are some of your safest bets.

Sustainable harvested seafood uses methods that protect the oceans natural supply and avoid harming other sea life in the process. Natural Resources Defense Council, Clean Fish, Marine Stewardship Council, and the EWG are resources you can trust when purchasing your seafood. Here in Cancun I have the benefit of being able to purchase my fish fresh from a local market. I always stick with smaller fish that have low mercury levels and use this as a guide:

MERCURY LEVELS IN FISH

HIGH	MEDIUM	LOW	
Bluefish	Bass (striped, black)	Arctic Cod	Perch (ocean)
Crab (blue)	Carp	Anchovies	Plaice
Grouper*	Cod (alaskan)	Butterfish	Pollock
Mackerel (king, spanish, gulf)	Croaker (white pacific)	Catfish	Salmon**
Marlin*	Halibut (pacific, atlantic)	Clam	(canned, fresh, wild)
Orange Roughy*	Lobster	Crab (domestic)	Sardine
Salmon**	Mahi Mahi	Crawfish/Crayfish	Scallop*
(farmed, atlantic)	Monkfish*	Croaker (atlantic)	Shad
Seabass (chilean)	Perch (freshwater)	Flounder*	Shrimp*
Shark*	Sablefish	Haddock (atlantic)	Sole
Swordfish*	Skate*	Hake	Squid
Tilefish Tuna	Snapper*	Herring	Tilapia
(ahi*, yellowfin*, bigeye, blue, canned albacore)	Tuna (canned chunk light, skipjack*)	Mackerel (n. atlantic, chub)	Trout
	Sea Trout	Mullet	Whitefish
		Oyster	Whiting

*OVERFISHED, ** MAY CONTAIN PCB'S - DATA FROM NRDC.ORG

Fair Trade and Rainforest Alliance

Fairtrade is the most recognized and trusted sustainability label in the world. Fairtrade changes the way trade works through better prices, decent working conditions and a fairer deal for farmers and workers in developing countries. The Fair Trade federation and World Fair Trade Organization are two groups committed to supporting fair trade principles through the supply chain. You can support sustainable farming practices by purchasing products with a Rainforest Alliance seal when shopping. The seal means that the certified product or ingredient was produced using methods that support the three pillars of sustainability: social, economic, and environmental. You can find their logo on their goods.

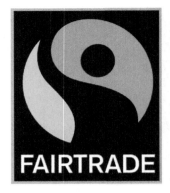

Clean Label Project

I learned of the Clean Label Project while I was researching baby and infant formulas for Zuri. Currently, the Food and Drug Administration (FDA) does not set specific limits on the amount of heavy metals in baby food. Metal contamination has been linked to the development of autism, ADHD and other neurological disorders. I know, unbelievably sad right? The good news is that times are changing thanks to the recent class-action lawsuits against big baby brands (yup, all your favorites, including Gerber, Beech-Nut, Earth's Best Organic, Parent's Choice, Plum Organics and Sprout Foods) whose products have been found to be tainted with toxic metals such as arsenic, lead, cadmium, and mercury. As of September 1, 2022, there are over 100 lawsuits pending and these products are still on store shelves. Which is why this US-based non-profit is worthy of the

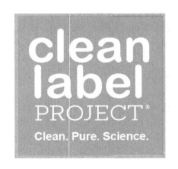

mention as they have a powerful mission of bringing truth and transparency to food and consumer product labeling. They're taking notice of by rewarding brands that are going above and beyond the minimal regulations required by the FDA. What stands out most about their mission is that they consider more than just the pathogen and microbiological contaminants and pay attention to the health consequences of exposure to heavy metals, pesticide residues, and plasticizers. Watch for their logos on the world's purest products and visit them online to source these products in a store near you.

Now that you know how to make smarter choices with label reading you're all set to be a conscious consumer and see through those products that, thanks to sneaky marketing, look healthy when they're not.

SHOULD YOU GO GLUTEN-FREE?

Going gluten-free isn't just a trend, there is research to back up the health benefits. The number of gluten-related digestive problems has skyrocketed.

My work with clients over the years has given prominence to the correlation between gut issues and gluten. Gluten, the protein in wheat, barley, and rye, has been found to damage the lining of the gut. So even if you aren't showing signs of intolerance, your gut and entire body would be in better condition without it. A healthy gut contributes to a strong immune system, heart health, brain health, improved mood, healthy sleep, and effective digestion. Additionally, it may help prevent some cancers and degenerative and autoimmune diseases. If you need another reason to eliminate gluten, most industrial wheat is sprayed with glyphosate (also known as Roundup) at harvest to exfoliate the plant and make wheat easier to harvest. This is why we find high levels of glyphosate in breakfast cereals. A little roundup with your cornflakes? Imagine giving this to your children. No thanks, never ever!

You may have thought about going gluten-free before but dreaded the thought of eliminating some of your favorite foods. Removing gluten is less complicated than it seems. To clarify any confusion, gluten-free is not synonymous with carb-free. Going gluten-free means you replace gluten with plant-based, complex carbohydrates. It's not meant to be low-carb or restrictive. Gluten-free diets should be rich in these healthy, complex carbohydrates which include starchy vegetables like potatoes, sweet potatoes, rice, pumpkin, and carrots. All fruits and vegetables are your friends when living a gluten-free lifestyle. Throughout the pages of this book, you'll find my favorite grain and gluten-free options: coconut flour, almond flour, chickpea flour, cassava flour, gluten-free oats (all of which I use to make wraps, bread, and tortillas), and oat flour, sweet potato, and wild, basmati, or black rice. I don't include a single recipe containing gluten! You'll also find my favorite pseudo-grains: buckwheat, quinoa, millet, and amaranth. These options are all low glycemic, nutrient-dense, and gut-friendly. One of the most important qualities of these carbs is they contain resistant starch. So starch is not absorbed and digested, and it won't cause a rise in blood sugar. One final benefit is that it feeds gut bacteria.

Eliminating gluten can have profound positive health impacts: reduced inflammation, weight loss, skin improvements, and better gut health. Still skeptical? Try eliminating it completely from your diet for a month and see how different you feel. You'll discover this is a better way to see how effective this change is than any blood or food intolerance test from a Doctor.

You want to watch out for products labeled 'gluten-free.' A plethora of these products are loaded with sugar and artificial ingredients—often more than the processed foods they're trying to replace. Gluten-free cookies and brownies are still cookies and brownies, and they may be even worse in terms of sugar content and glycemic index. Read those labels well with your new skills!

All things considered, even if you don't suffer from intolerance, inflammation, or digestive issues from gluten, I still recommend limiting your consumption of these items. And unless you have Celiac Disease, which only about 1 percent of the population has, you don't have to give up gluten completely. Yes, I love a serving of sourdough bread (yum—warm bread!) and ice cream. I just consciously choose to enjoy these items, in moderation, on occasion, and ensure I don't overconsume them—I'll pay the consequences. Learn what your threshold is and honor it.

Created by the amazing female body, breast milk delivers nutrients for our babies' nourishment, development, and growth. As we grow up, dairy expands to include milk, cheese, and yogurt. Its role in adulthood is heavily questioned. Although it's an excellent source of calcium, protein, and nutrients, many people don't tolerate it. Adults don't produce lactase (the enzyme that breaks down lactose). 75% of the population is considered lactose intolerant. Dairy intolerance symptoms include bloating, gas, brain fog, and nasal drip. There is also evidence that supports that dairy may contribute to acne and eczema and can be a main contributor to menstrual cycle-related pain.

However, quality is an important factor. Poor quality dairy is full of hormones that can cause fat gain and cancer. Personally, if I consume any amount of poor-quality dairy, I immediately start bloating and experience nasal drip. I don't have the same reaction to high-quality dairy. My weekly dairy consumption ranges from two to four servings of high-quality dairy spread throughout the week. My main dairy choices are ghee (clarified butter) for cooking and baking, yogurt, cheese, and cottage cheese (for my ah-maaazing cottage cheese pancakes check out page 114).

In my years of working with over a thousand people, I've observed that, especially when consumed in excess, it doesn't sit well with most people. For many women eliminating dairy can dramatically improve period pain, heavy periods, endometriosis, acne, and PMS. If you're not sure if you're intolerant, I advise the same thing as I did above with gluten. Eliminate it completely from your diet for a month and see how you feel. This gives you some time to try the healthy, dairy-free milk alternatives on the market. You may end up discovering you feel better without milk. Making the swap isn't as difficult as you may think (plus my recipes make it easy!).

My Tips for Choosing High-Quality Dairy

Choose Non-GMO and Organic for higher quality, nutrients, flavor, and consistency.

Go for Grass-fed. This is particularly important when buying full fat. The second best choice is pasture-raised.

Go for the Goat. It may be better tolerated as it contains A2 casein instead of the inflammatory A1 type found in conventional cow dairy.

Choose Regular Fat over Low Fat. Most low-fat options have added sugar while full-fat dairy is loaded with healthy fat-soluble vitamins. Read your labels! If you choose a low-fat option to reduce your calories, be sure you choose plain varieties with no added sugar and add your own sweetener like stevia or sugar-free syrup with fruit.

Go for Greek. Greek contains more protein than regular yogurt. If you can't find organic Greek, you can add protein powder to plain, organic yogurt, and voila, you've just created your own Greek yogurt.

Go for Ghee over Butter or Margarine. Ghee, or clarified butter, has all the milk proteins removed and is usually well tolerated. This is a great heat-stable fat for cooking plus the flavor is so much better.

Look for lactose-free options. If you prefer, organic and lactose-free is a great combination. Watch for added sugars and sneaky ingredients like gums, flavors, and fillers. I find these creamy, delicious, and great for smoothies and as a creamer in coffee.

Be Wary of Vegan Cheese. If you're purchasing vegan cheese, read the labels carefully for added ingredients like unhealthy oils and fillers. Sometimes when animal products are cut out, they may be replaced with unhealthy plant-based products and dairy-free cheese can fall into this vegan junk food trap. I have yet to find a vegan cheese to approve. My go-to cheese is organic goat cheese.

What You Need To Know About Dairy-Free Milk

Back in the day, when you were buying milk, you only had a few choices based on the fat content you wanted: whole milk, 2%, or skim. Nowadays, our grocery aisles are packed with a flock of non-dairy or plant-based milk made from nuts, legumes, seeds, and grains. Soy milk, almond milk, cashew milk, hemp milk, coconut milk, oat milk, flax milk, rice milk…there's no shortage of substitutes. The questions I'm most often asked are, do these substitutes fully replace the nutrients in cow's milk, and what is the best choice to make?

When we talk about living dairy-free, calcium concerns frequently arise. But it's important to know that calcium is abundant in our food supply. It's naturally found in many foods and is also added via fortification in products like our dairy-free milk alternatives. Plant milks aren't naturally rich in calcium and vitamin D so it's best to choose a brand that is fortified with both as most companies are now. For example, one cup of skim milk offers 300 mg of calcium per cup. As a reference, according to the National Institute of Health, the RDA (recommended dietary allowance) for calcium for children 1 to 3 years old is 700 mg per day. This increases to 1000 mg from 4 to 8 years old and up to 1300 mg per day until the age of 18 when it drops slightly to 1000 mg for most of our lives.

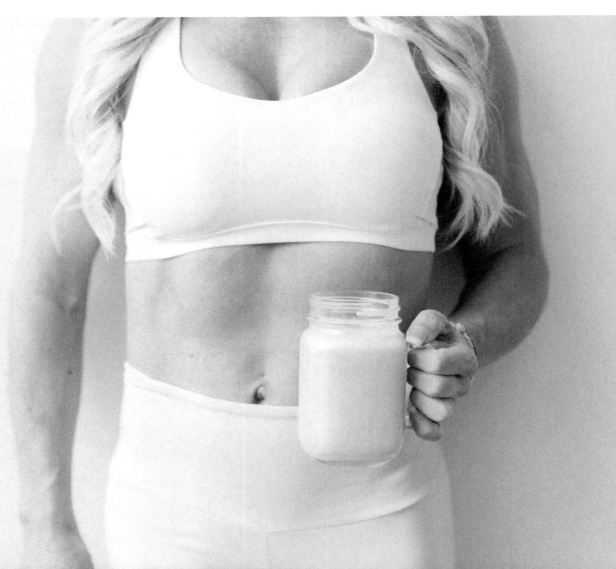

My Tips for Choosing a Dairy-Free Milk Alternative:

Non-GMO and Organic—quality counts.

Unsweetened—always over sweetened.

Fortification—most brands are now fortified (adding micronutrients to food and beverages) with calcium and vitamin D, vitamin B-12, and other vitamins. If you want to reap the full benefits of plant-based milk, then you need to check if it's fortified. Making your milk at home? Understand that you'll need to get those nutrients from other food sources. Finally, plant-based milk for your children should always be fortified.

Avoid thickeners and additives—try your best to avoid these items when possible. These are ingredients like carrageenan, carboxymethylcellulose, and polysorbate-80. They may have inflammatory effects on the gut and cause digestion issues.

Avoid added oils—canola, sunflower or grape seed. These are inflammatory and, in this instance, the least amount of ingredients is best.

Avoid rice milk—it may contain high levels of arsenic.

Limit emulsifiers—you'll often find food-grade gums such as gellan gum, xanthan gum, guar gum, and locust bean gum used as thickening agents in non-dairy milk. They may cause gastrointestinal distress so if you notice a sensitivity to them then avoid these items.

Depending on your body goals, you may glance at the calories as well. There is a lot of high-quality vegan milk on the market that is between 25-40 calories per cup. You can make your own at home too!

In our home, we use a variety of organic, dairy-free milk alternatives. I haven't consumed milk from a cow for over two decades due to the added sugars, hormones, and higher calorie content. We also feel healthier using dairy-free milk. My preference is almond or macadamia for my shakes and coconut creamer or lactose-free for my coffee since it has a creamer taste. For my daughter, I use organic, fortified oat milk. It's the highest in calories among dairy-free milk. Dairy-free milk is lower in protein (except for soy milk); however, I fill in this gap with other protein sources like eggs, cheese, lean meats, and a plant-based complete nutrition powder (I love the American brand ELSE because their products meet the highest standards; they're certified organic and undergo testing for over 400 contaminants and heavy metals). Apart from protein, most store-bought plant milk is fortified with the same vitamins and minerals that you would find in dairy milk. If you're choosing dairy-free milk for your baby check with your pediatrician to ensure you're meeting their RDI's for vitamins and minerals.

You'll find my recipes make removing dairy simple as they call for dairy-free milk. Plant-based milk is an excellent milk alternative because it's dairy-free, is better for our planet, and is typically lower in calories, sugar, and saturated fat than cow's milk.

All things considered, going dairy free is a personal choice. If you do choose to consume any dairy, I recommend going with quality dairy, consuming in moderation, and always based on how you feel.

Life is certainly a little sweeter with sugar. However, I know I don't need to tell you that the levels of sugar our society currently consumes are a direct reflection of our global chronic health concerns. The average American consumes over 70 g of sugar each day—that's 17 whole teaspoons. That translates into about 57 pounds of sugar consumed per person, each year!

That oh-so-sweet sugar causes glucose and insulin levels to spike and plummet. The fluctuation of these levels can cause fat storage and leave you feeling hungry soon after you eat, causing you to eat more. This cycle can lead to fat gain over time, in addition to mood changes, poor memory function, brain fog, and other cognitive issues. Excessive sugar consumption is playing a major role in overall health. I say 'excessive' because a little sugar isn't going to kill you. While it's true that less is better, that doesn't mean you can't have any at all. It's all about—yup, you guessed it—moderation. We now know excess sugar contributes to an increased risk of diabetes, obesity, and heart disease. We know it suppresses immune function, leads to chromium deficiency, accelerates aging, causes tooth decay and gum disease (which can lead to heart disease), affects cognition in children, decreases 'good' gut bacteria (which can lead to inflammation), and takes the place of important nutrients.

Sugar also has been associated with addiction. It's highly toxic and detoxing is not easy. The struggle is real, and your willpower will be tested to the max. Sugar lights up the addiction center in the brain like heroin or cocaine, so when we're talking about sugar addiction properties being similar to cocaine, I mean that sugar's cyclical bursts of serotonin and beta-endorphin are no joke—brains can rewire themselves to crave sugar—and you can end up with real withdrawal symptoms when you don't get enough of the sweet stuff. The amount of hidden sugars in food products is one of the main culprits. Considering how much hidden sugar there is in our food supply, I think it's safe to say that most of us have suffered from sugar addiction, intentionally or not, at one time or another in our life (me included!). Did you know there are over 50 different names that manufacturers use for sugar to disguise it in your food?

Here are 30 of them:

1.	corn sweetener	16.	florida crystals
2.	ethyl maltol	17.	cane sugar
3.	corn syrup	18.	crystalline fructose
4.	dextrose	19.	evaporated cane juice
5.	fructose	20.	corn syrup solids
6.	fruit juice concentrates	21.	malt syrup
7.	glucose	22.	barley malt
8.	high-fructose corn syrup	23.	agave nectar
9.	invert sugar	24.	rice syrup
10.	lactose	25.	caramel
11.	maltose	26.	panocha
12.	malt syrup	27.	muscovado
13.	raw sugar	28.	molasses
14.	sucrose	29.	treacle
15.	sugar syrup	30.	carob syrup

When I visited Canada recently, I was shocked to discover how much 'hidden' added sugar there is in different products. I found added sugar in so-called 'healthy and organic' products like oat milk, yogurt, and an organic bean salad in a jar. In Mexico, it's not as prevalent as we definitely have cleaner, healthier options, but there is still added sugar in some foods. Manufacturers are getting away with it and many consumers are straight-up addicted to certain brands for this reason. Bottom line—even if it's organic rice syrup or cane sugar, it's still sugar. Take the time to read your labels!

The Glycemic Index and Glycemic Load

Picture a roller coaster with loads of ups and downs. That's what your blood sugar and insulin levels look like over the course of a day. The highs that follow meals and snacks drop to lows later on. For optimal health, you want to learn to eat so your blood sugar levels look more like a kiddie coaster with gentle ups and downs. How do we accomplish this? A little system called the glycemic index (GI). This is an awesome tool to promote better blood sugar management. The GI measures how quickly and how high a particular food raises your blood sugar level. Food is classified as low, medium, or high glycemic food and ranked on a scale of 0-100. The closer a food compares to pure glucose (which is given a ranking of 100), the more likely it is that it will raise blood sugar levels. As we know, large vacillations in blood sugar can put our bodies in fat storage mode and create dips in our energy. Using the GI as a guide of what you're putting on your plate, in turn, helps you enhance fat loss, decrease your blood sugar levels, and reduce your cholesterol.

Several factors influence the GI of a food:

- **nutrient composition**
- **cooking method**
- **ripeness (a ripe bananas GI is double that of an unripe banana)**
- **processing**

The lower the GI of a specific food, the less it may affect your blood sugar levels:

GI ratings are classified into three levels:

- **Low: 55 or less***
- **Medium: 56-69**
- **High: 70 or above (sugar has a ranking of 100)**
*75% of your food should fall under the low category.

The following are my favorite healthy and low GI foods:

- **Fruits: Granny Smith apples, berries, pears, grapes, kiwi oranges, lemons, limes, grapefruit**
- **Non-starchy vegetables: broccoli, cauliflower, carrots, spinach, tomatoes**
- **Whole grains: black, red, and white quinoa, black rice, brown basmati rice, wild rice, barley, sweet potato with the skin on, whole grain sourdough and sprouted grain bread (these are not gluten-free and I consume occasionally), buckwheat, farro, amaranth, large flake or steel cut oats**
- **Legumes: lentils, black beans, chickpeas, kidney beans**
- **Others: dark chocolate, yogurt**

Although there are no strictly 'off-limits' foods, reduce your intake of foods with a high GI because they are almost always refined carbohydrates with most fiber and nutrition stripped away.

Foods with a high GI include:
- **Bread: white bread, bagels, naan, pita bread**
- **Rice: white rice, jasmine rice, arborio rice**
- **Cereals: instant oats, breakfast cereals**
- **Pasta and noodles: lasagna, spaghetti, ravioli, macaroni, fettuccine**
- **Starchy vegetables: mashed potatoes, potatoes, French fries**
- **Baked goods: cake, doughnuts, cookies, croissants, muffins**
- **Snacks: chocolate, crackers, microwave popcorn, chips, pretzels**
- **Sugar-sweetened beverages: soda, fruit juice, sports drinks**

If you're currently consuming a lot of high-GI foods, don't think of it as 'giving them up,' but rather 'replacing' these foods with healthier alternatives (say hello to all my healthy desserts!). Start with 1-2 items until you've been able to replace most of these foods in your diet.

One more measure to consider is the glycemic load (GL). While the glycemic index only determines how quickly a carbohydrate is digested and converted into glucose in the bloodstream, the glycemic load takes into account how much of the carbohydrate we consume in one sitting. A high GI ranking isn't the entire story and doesn't automatically mean it's going to be an unhealthy choice. This is where the GL comes into play. Portion size is key.

One thing I wish I had known sooner is you can eat natural, higher GI foods in small quantities and combine them with other foods to moderate their glycemic impact. For example, a naturally sweet food like a date or banana (moderate GI) paired with a bit of protein will modulate your blood sugar response, preventing those deadly spikes and crashes that set you up for cravings, constant hunger, fat gain, and diabetes. Super cool, right? I think I avoided bananas for close to a decade! As you can see, the GI is valuable, but it's only part of the story when it comes to how your body responds to an entire meal.

Use the GI/GL as guides, but there's no need to obsess over numbers. Make an overall effort to remember which foods are higher on the spectrum. Focus on consuming mostly low to moderate GI foods. Eat healthy portion sizes. Slow down when chewing. Add cinnamon and as much fiber as possible to reduce the glycemic load of each meal and have a steady source of fuel. And, if you need some sweetness, combine naturally sweet food with lower GI food to minimize your blood sugar response.

How Sugar Stores Fat

Sugar is energy. It's like the gas in your car. When you fill-up your car, you use some of that gasoline as you leave the station, but the rest is stored in your tank. The same principle applies to eating sugar. Your body either uses it immediately or stores it for later in your muscles and your liver. And remember that when talking about sugar here, I mean carbohydrates. Everything from table sugar to red pepper has some sugar in it.

But, as I discussed in the carbohydrates section, your 'tank,' muscles and liver, can only store a limited amount of glycogen—about a day's worth. Glycogen is a pretty short-term energy strategy.

Now, your brain is a huge consumer of energy—think of it as the gas guzzler—it uses 20% of your energy. We also know that the brain is pretty important for daily life—nothing better than a day when your brain is ignited! But without another source of fuel—additional eaten sugar or another form of storage—your brain could quickly run out of gas.

You know what this feels like. Does the word 'hangry' ring any bells?

So we need to effectively store energy if we want more than just survival—we want to function at our best with a steady supply of fuel. Unlike our car, we have a second strategy for long-term energy needs—we have the practically unlimited ability to store sugar as fat. Sugar that doesn't fit in the tank can be stored as fat. Fat is a much longer-term energy strategy. This was great when we needed to live off fat stores back when we hunted and gathered our food, but we certainly don't do that now.

These foods introduce large doses of sugar into your bloodstream, quickly. Blood sugar levels act as a signal to the pancreas to produce insulin—a hormone that converts food into glucose. It tells the cells to open up and let sugar in to be converted to glycogen and stored in the muscles and liver. When that's full, the excess sugar is converted to triglycerides and stored in the muscles and fat tissue to be used later. If you don't eat a lot of carbohydrates, you can use this energy pretty easily. If carbohydrates are a regular and large part of your diet, it's much more difficult.

If your sugar intake gets out of control, it can lead to a negative cascade effect. The more sugar you eat, the more insulin you release. And, because the purpose of insulin is to help store energy away, the more sugar you eat, the less access you have to stored energy—its job is to store sugar and keep it there (i.e., not to let it out).

Again, excess sugar is stored as fat and cannot be used to fill energy demands due to the excess insulin circulating in the bloodstream over an extended period. So, in the end, you'll get hungry for more sugar when your body requires energy.

By choosing foods that do not trigger this cycle, you'll simply use what you have stored—it won't be locked away by circulating insulin. You'll have good metabolic flexibility. Your body will be able to switch between breaking down carbs or fat easily, and you'll have better weight maintenance, increased energy levels, improved sleep, optimized workout performance, and improved overall health. So, it's not necessary to cut out carbs from your diet for lean body composition. Instead, learn which types of carbohydrates are the most beneficial along with the correct portions.

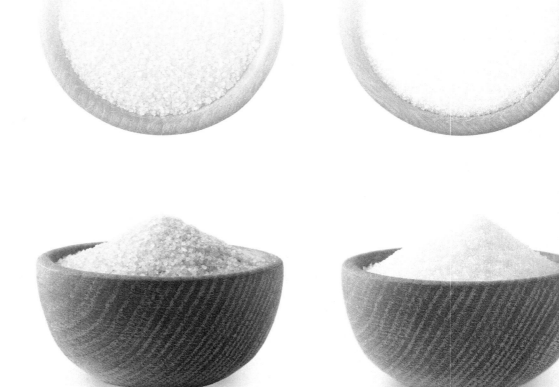

Sugar and Hormones

Sugar impacts our hunger and satiety hormones. I'm sure at some point you've experienced such an uncontrollable surge in your appetite, that you just don't feel satiated no matter how much you eat and all you want is sugar! I experienced this after every competition when I would introduce a swell of sugar into my body after restricting it for so long. This is a horrible, vicious cycle that starts from consuming high-in-sugar processed foods in excess.

Meet leptin—the satiety or appetite-regulating hormone—and ghrelin—the hunger hormone.

The way the first works is that when leptin rises, your appetite diminishes. Leptin is crucial in controlling how much you eat. When your brain receives the leptin signal, it says 'I'm not starving, I don't need to eat so much.' Your body can then relax, menstruate, have a baby, build strong bones, and have a normal immune system. Without the leptin signal, the brain says 'I'm starving, I need to reduce my expenditure and increase my food intake to source energy and be able to make more leptin'

Leptin regulates your metabolism and the fat breakdown rate. As leptin levels rise, your metabolic rate increases. As leptin levels fall, your metabolism slows.

Leptin levels can be maintained through a proper diet. It's important to have balanced leptin regulation—not too much or too little. If you're constantly putting yourself into a calorie deficit (this is for my chronic low-calorie dieters!), you will lower your leptin levels and slow your metabolic rate. Slowing down your metabolism is what makes it difficult to lose body fat. This is why we don't eat 'less' to lose 'fat.' Hormone and metabolism health are indicators of how easily your body will achieve a goal (fat loss, muscle gain, performance, etc.). Most new clients who start working with me have been yo-yo dieting on and off for years, resulting in an unhealthy and slow metabolism. It can take anywhere from 1-6 months to repair a damaged metabolism once following an individualized nutrition and movement program. Too much leptin can also be detrimental. Overweight people have large amounts of leptin, but their brains are not getting the signal to stop eating. This can result in weight gain that is difficult to lose because insulin blocks leptin (leptin resistance) by telling your fat cells to store energy or hold onto body fat and prevent you from losing fat.

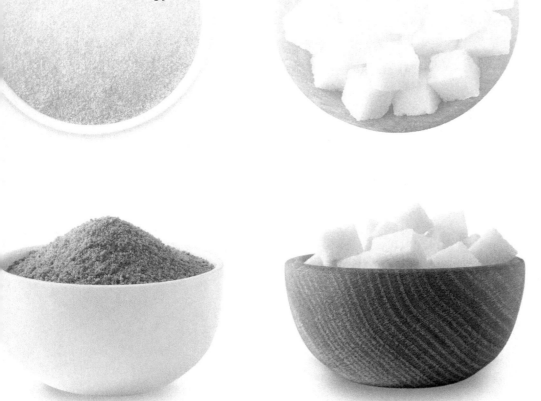

Some simple and effective ways to keep your leptin levels regulated are to get enough fiber, eat optimal protein (especially with breakfast), consume complex carbohydrates, avoid severe calorie restriction, get more sleep, take omega-3 essential fatty acids, and perform H.I.I.T (high-intensity interval training).

There's also insulin, the hormone that regulates most metabolic processes. It's well documented that excess sugar consumption is a key driver of many of the most serious modern diseases. Metabolic syndrome (obesity, type II diabetes, heart disease) is increasingly common, and up to one-third of U.S. adults have it. This is linked to a condition called insulin resistance. Normally, your digestive system breaks down food you eat into sugar. Insulin is a hormone made by your pancreas that helps sugar enter your cells to be used as fuel. In people with insulin resistance, cells don't respond normally to insulin. Glucose can't enter the cells as easily. This may be scary because as a result, your blood sugar levels rise even as your body churns out more and more insulin to try to lower your blood sugar. This is where everyone's body is unique. Someone with insulin resistance will process carbs very differently than someone healthy. If this is you, don't lose hope. It can be improved. I've helped many of my clients decrease and even reverse insulin resistance with a customized approach to whole food nutrition and a healthy lifestyle. The recipes in this book are a great place to start.

The Best Natural Sweeteners

I'm all about 'sweeting responsibly' and the great news is, you can! There are some great options to naturally sweeten food that can add nutrition without detrimental effects on blood sugar and hormones and without exposing our bodies to the chemicals found in synthetic sugar substitutes.

I know this variety of sugar substitutes nowadays can be confusing, so I've given you the low down on my top natural sweeteners:

Monk Fruit Powder

This is my sweetener of choice. I love getting my sweeteners from sources as close to nature as possible, so monk fruit is also a great option I keep on hand. The extract is 150-200 times sweeter than sugar and contains zero calories, zero carbohydrates, zero sodium, and zero fat. Most noticeably, it doesn't raise blood glucose levels, making it a popular option for diabetics and health-conscious foodies like me. The sweetener is derived from the native Chinese plant, and many properties have been used in Traditional Chinese Medicine for centuries. Monk fruit powder is often available at your local health food store, so if you're looking to branch out this is a wonderful option. Read your label and watch for additives. You want to purchase pure monk fruit sweetener.

Stevia

Stevia is a sugar substitute made from the leaves of the stevia plant from South America. Stevia is a nonnutritive sweetener that doesn't spike blood sugar levels. It's 100-300 times sweeter than sugar. It's important to note that it is zero-calorie but it also lacks any good nutrients. Many of the readily available alternatives are packed with artificial additives so make sure you read your labels to purchase the pure form, which has a bit of a bitter aftertaste but it's free of any sugar alcohol's or artificial ingredients. I don't use stevia for baking but I love a dash in my coffee or to add sweetness to drinks. Try to avoid the blends and go with pure stevia. Most often this is found in drops.

Maple Syrup

Growing up in Canada this was a staple topping! In it's purest form, when taken from the sap of the maple tree, it's taste is enough to sweeten even the most bitter of dishes with a lovely homely flavor. Not only is it a beautiful sweetener, but when enjoyed in balance it can actually have some incredible health benefits. It contains calcium, potassium, iron, zinc, and manganese, alongside at least 24 antioxidants. Plus, some active compounds in maple syrup have been shown to help reduce the growth of cancer cells and may slow down the breakdown of carbohydrates in the digestive tract. Grade A Very Dark will be better for you. It has more antioxidants and mineral content than the lighter colors. And be cautious, the pure form isn't to be confused with maple-flavored syrup, which is sugar syrup with chemically derived maple flavors. There are naturally flavored options that are sweetened with stevia on the market but check your labels to confirm that they aren't any unwanted additives. I've used stevia or monk fruit syrups in my recipes to keep the sugar lower; however, if you prefer, you can use a combination of pure maple syrup with stevia syrup for a richer flavor and more nutritious creation. And if you want to use the real thing, go for it with the 'a little goes a long way mindset' as 1 tbsp yields 14g of sugar. All grades of maple syrup and white table sugar have roughly the same amount of sugar, when comparing equal portions of each.

Coconut Sugar

A simple swap for any sweet recipe is coconut sugar. This is still to be consumed in moderation, but carries a lot more nutrients than refined white sugar. It is made from the dehydrated sap of the coconut palm and retains nutrients such as the minerals iron, zinc, calcium, and potassium, along with some short-chain fatty acids like polyphenols and antioxidants. This sugar is nutritive but it does increase blood sugar.

Dates

This fruit is one of the most nutrient-rich sources of natural sugars and can be used in anything from baking and smoothies to salads and syrups. This high-fiber fruit is perhaps best known for its powerful digestive properties, but it's good for so much more than that. Dates have a widespread nutrient profile and are packed with various antioxidants, alongside helping regulate cholesterol levels, strengthening the nervous system, and improving bone health. Again, they still need to be consumed in moderation as 1 cup of chopped dates yields 93g of sugar. I love using them in my overnight oats - be sure to check out the Triple Layer Salted Caramel Oats on page 137.

Raw Honey

This option is a naturally delicious syrupy option and I love it for the abundance of health and antimicrobial benefits it offers. As honey becomes more widely used for health purposes, emerging studies are confirming what we already know; that the antibacterial benefits are extremely potent. This sugar is nutritive but does increase blood sugar therefore use this sparingly. Because it's an animal byproduct, honey is technically not vegan - so may not be a suitable option for all. We also need to be cautious of sustainability as our growing demand for bees has created a honey bee decline. Supporting local, sustainable beekeepers is one of the best decisions you can make.

Unsulfured Molasses

Molasses made from ripe sugar cane are called unsulfured molasses because it has no additives. If green, unripe sugarcane is used, it is treated with sulfur dioxide first to preserve it. It can leave a chemical taste in the mouth, so I recommend looking for unsulfured molasses whenever possible. This sugar is nutritive but does increase blood sugar. This is a good option for your Mom's Christmas gingersnap cookie recipe.

Sugar Alcohols

Sugar alcohols have half the calories of sugar and have a slight influence on your blood sugars, but overall, they're safe to include as part of a balanced diet if you're not over consuming them. Unlike sugar, sugar alcohols are not absorbed or digested fully so overconsumption can cause bloating, gas, upset stomach and diarrhea. They're not going to kill you but everyone digests these differently so monitor bloating and gas when you consume them. They're low in calories and carbs, but not free of them. You'll want to subtract half of the grams of sugar alcohol listed on the food label from the total grams of carbohydrate. Common sugar alcohols include Xylitol, Erythritol, Sorbitol and Maltitol. You'll often find them blended with stevia or monk fruit sweetener and in baked goods, candy and gums labeled 'sugar-free.'

Allulose

Allulose is a sugar you'll see popping up in products lately. It's classified as a 'rare sugar' because it is naturally present in only a few foods. Wheat, figs and raisins all contain it.

Like glucose and fructose, allulose is a monosaccharide, or single sugar. It has the same chemical formula as fructose, but is arranged differently. This difference in structure prevents your body from processing allulose the way it processes fructose.

It is about 70% as sweet as sugar, which is similar to the sweetness of erythritol.

It doesn't provide much nutrition as 70-84% of the allulose you consume is absorbed into your blood from your digestive tract, it is eliminated in the urine without being used as fuel. It's been shown to resist fermentation by your gut bacteria, minimizing the likelihood of bloating, gas or other digestive problems. And the good news is it doesn't raise blood sugar or insulin levels. Allulose also provides only 0.2-0.4 calories per gram, or about 1/10 the calories of table sugar. In addition, early research suggests that allulose has anti-inflammatory properties, and may help prevent obesity and reduce the risk of chronic disease.

Agave didn't make my list - you may be wondering why. I don't use it as it's basically a condensed fructose syrup, with minimal nutritional value due to being highly processed. When it comes to sugar alternatives you've got far better options!

Avoid Artificial Sweeteners

The name gives it away. Artificial sweeteners are toxic chemicals that your body doesn't recognize, and therefore can't respond to. As a result, these concoctions create metabolic changes, disrupt healthy gut bacteria, add stress to the liver, and might even create more fat gain than eating real sugar by stimulating hunger hormones. These can also alter gut flora, leading to inconsistent blood sugar levels. Diet soft drinks fit into this category—often seen as a healthy beverage as they contain very few if any, carbs or calories—but they aren't a good substitute at all for sugar-sweetened drinks. The artificial sweeteners in diet soft drinks, such as aspartame, Sucralose, acesulfame K, and saccharin can trigger an insulin response, causing your body to store fat instead of using it for fuel. They may also alter sweet taste receptors, making it harder to appreciate the natural sweetness of real food. Remember to check your labels since artificial sweeteners are also commonly found in dairy products like yogurt, snack foods, and sugar-free candies.

Choose to avoid them and drink water, tea, or naturally sweetened drinks that contain no carbs and are better for your health. You can make your water more exciting by adding slices of fresh fruit (grapefruit or strawberries), veggies (cucumber or celery), herbs (mint, basil, or lavender), or other combinations. Don't miss my 'Mocktail' chapter as well which features some of my favorite go-to healthy drinks.

The takeaway on sugar: it's a balance, and you never want to feel like sugar is off-limits—unless you're detoxing from it. You're going to find the longer you have sugar out of your life, the less you want it. This is the 'sweet spot' (pun intended) you're aiming for. Your body will ask for more of the healthy stuff simply because you're creating balanced, whole food meals that include natural sources of sugar like fruits, eating before you get hungry (catching that blood sugar crash!), and staying consistent with it! Use the nutritive sugar alternatives I've shared above and my healthy dessert recipes to help you curb those cravings without adding calories. You've got this.

Choosing a Protein Powder

If you're looking for a convenient way to boost protein in your healthy and lean diet, you need protein powder in your life! It's not just for bodybuilders. Anyone, at any age, who wants to optimize their health can benefit from a good protein powder. Muscle mass decreases approximately 3-8% per decade after the age of 30 (which is called sarcopenia). This rate of decline is even higher after the age of 60. My 71-year-old father adds a scoop of protein to his oats every morning to set himself up for the win when it comes to meeting his daily protein requirements! Protein powders are convenient and tasty. Most importantly, a quality protein shake or smoothie bowl made from whole food ingredients (like those in my recipes!) can benefit your health in so many ways. BUT, you guessed it, all protein powders aren't created equal. Before I dive in, let's first clarify what protein powder is.

What is Protein Powder?

Protein powders are powdered forms of protein that come from plants (soybeans, peas, rice, oats, potatoes, or hemp), eggs, milk (casein or whey protein), and even insects—yes, insects have recently been identified as a more sustainable protein-dense food source and may represent a viable alternative to conventional animal-derived proteins! Protein powders are food-based; however, they're considered dietary supplements due to different manufacturing aspects. Currently, the FDA leaves it up to the manufacturer to evaluate product safety and labeling. This becomes an issue because the supplement industry is poorly regulated in most countries. It's up to us as consumers to educate ourselves and make health-conscious choices. Protein powders are one of the most heavily contaminated products on the market. Earlier this year the Clean Label Project released a report about toxins in protein powders. Researchers screened 134 products for 130 types of toxins and found that many protein powders contain heavy metals (lead, arsenic, cadmium, and mercury), bisphenol-A (BPA, which is used to make plastic), pesticides, or other contaminants with links to cancer and other health conditions. Some toxins were present in significant quantities. One protein powder contained 25 times the allowed limit of BPA. (You can see this study at www.cleanlabelproject.org).

You can see why it's important to ignore all the marketing hype on the face of the package and head straight for the ingredients list, nutrition facts, and certifications. Purchase organic when possible. It may cost more, but your health is worth it. Additionally, the flavor and consistency of organic (and grass-fed if it's whey) are unsurpassable. Always look at the ingredients. Do you recognize all of them? Is it free of sugar, chemicals, additives, and fillers? Has it been third-party tested for heavy metals, pesticides, and other contaminants? Some protein powders are even product potency tested where these are compared to the information on the label.

Look for single ingredient powders and avoid the following ingredients for the highest quality protein and absorption:

> Gluten
> Dextrin/Maltodextrin
> Sugar and artificial sweeteners
> Any of the sneaky names I mentioned for hidden sugars
> Skim milk powders/milk solids
> Vegetable oils and fats
> Thickeners and gums
> Fillers

Avoid protein powders with added 'specialty' ingredients like mushroom powders or probiotics. You'll just pay more and not get the therapeutic dose required of the added ingredients.

For a more in-depth look at choosing a quality supplement read this article on my blog: https://ryallgraber.com/premiumsupplementfacts/

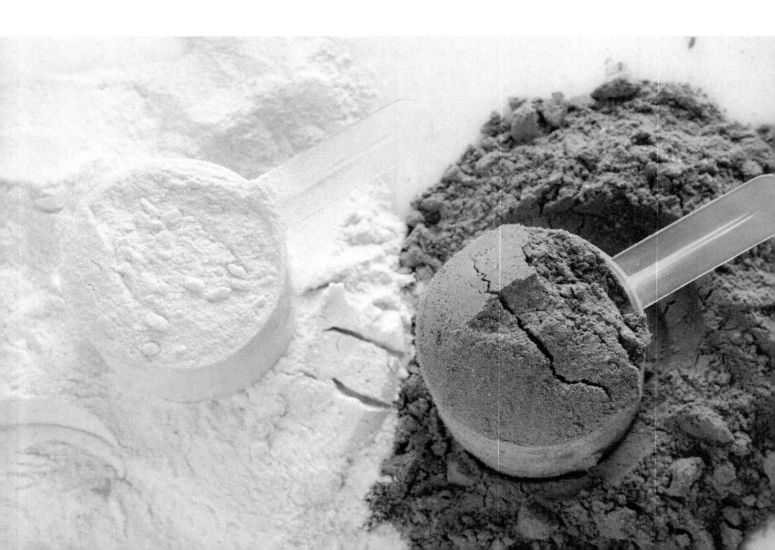

Which Protein Powder is Best for my Goals?

Choosing the right protein powder must suit your goals, dietary lifestyle, and health; and you've got to enjoy the taste, of course!

For weight loss, wellness, performance, and recovery I recommend any of the following types of protein powders as they contain optimal amino acid profiles. What's key is that you know when to use them and that you digest them well. You want to feel good while you're drinking it—and afterward!

Whey Protein—Whey protein is one of two proteins derived from dairy. During the manufacturing process, much of the lactose—or milk sugar—is filtered out, leaving a condensed product called whey protein concentrate. When this concentrate is further processed and filtered, you get whey protein isolate. Isolates have the highest percentage of pure protein and the lowest number of carbs per serving of any whey protein.

Whey is the optimal choice after exercise because it offers rapid digestion for post-workout recovery. To get that protein into your muscles quickly after a workout, you want to keep it simple by choosing just 3 ingredients: whey protein powder, water, and a small portion of fruit for some micronutrients and antioxidants. Plan to have a colorful, balanced meal for recovery as your hunger levels start to rise about an hour later.

Casein protein—Casein, the other milk protein, is also high quality but digested and absorbed much more slowly by your body than whey. This makes casein protein ideal for fasting periods, such as before bed or between meals. It's super thick to drink so either add extra liquid or whip it up with some almond milk for a delicious pudding.

If you have issues digesting lactose you may find that whey or casein protein aren't the best options for you. I struggled with this for years, but when I switched to an organic, grass-fed, single-ingredient, plain whey protein powder the bloating and gas disappeared. I keep referring to the importance of quality—but again, quality truly does matter! I add my own flavors by adding cocoa, matcha powder, vanilla extract, monk fruit sweetener, coffee, or stevia syrup. You can also mix them up. I love blending vegan and whey protein as a meal replacement to keep me fuller for longer. Plus, vegan powders can be really grainy and unappetizing so blending them with whey improves the taste and consistency.

Plant-based—Plant-based protein powders are derived from a variety of sources including pea, hemp, pumpkin seed, brown rice, soy, chia, and flax. They offer an alternative to animal-based powders (like whey and collagen). They're a bit higher in carbs, naturally higher in fiber, and are nutrient-dense than dairy protein powder. They're slower digesting, so they make a perfect meal replacement option at any time. Manufacturers frequently add sugar to improve taste, so read your labels carefully!

I'm often asked about the plant-based protein, soy, and although many people avoid eating soy protein due to its phytoestrogen content—concerned that this compound can disrupt natural hormone levels and promote breast cancer or affect male reproductive hormones (which current evidence does not support). I recommend avoiding soy because most soy foods are GMO. If you're going to choose a soy protein powder or consume any soy product, look for non-GMO and certified organic labels.

Egg Protein—Eggs are one of the most nutritious foods you can eat. This is a great non-dairy option if you're having difficulty digesting whey. I suggest using an egg powder that contains both the white and the yolk to get the full spectrum of nutrients. Perfect for an anytime, meal replacement that's low carb and medium-digesting.

Collagen Protein—An excellent addition to a healthy diet due to its added benefits such as promoting healthy skin and joints. The 5 types of collagen that are mainstream and seen in many collagen supplements are I, II, III, V, and X. But, there are more types in our bodies, possibly up to 28 (there's a lot of debate and differing research as the science around collagen continues). The human body needs different types of collagen for various functions in distinct parts. Some collagen types, like Type I, may improve skin quality and elasticity, strengthen nails, and help to grow healthier hair, additionally, it can help to rebuild your muscles, eyes, ligaments, bones, and spine. Others, like Type II, are good for stretching in multiple directions (ligaments, organs). When it comes to collagen supplements, most will be sourced from just beef and contain Type I & III. A multi collagen will offer all 5 types (I, II, III, V, & X) because it's sourced from beef, chicken, fish, and eggshell membrane. It's worth noting that collagen protein isn't a complete protein as it's missing one essential amino acid (tryptophan). I would not rely on this as your sole protein source. I suggest using this in addition to your other complete protein sources.

Psst. Looking for a great way to elevate your Joe? Mix it with coconut milk for the most awesome coffee creamer or pre-purchase it as a combination product. Unlike other powders, it mixes well into any hot liquid.

Insect protein—Recently, insect protein has hit the marketplace. Many countries in Asia, Oceania, Africa, and Latin America utilize insects as a major protein source. Using insects can potentially solve problems related to the conventional food-supply chain, including global water, land, and energy deficits and researchers generally agree that insects are extremely rich in protein, fat, and vitamins and may have prebiotic benefits. I personally haven't tried it so can't comment on the taste but if you are choosing an insect protein, I would ensure that it is non-GMO and follows safe manufacturing principles. For sure this is a protein to watch! Now, I know I ate that scorpion in Beijing and crickets in Mexico, but I would rather get my protein from other sources. If eating insects appeals to you, go for it, grasshopper!

Once you've decided on your protein powder(s), it's important to understand that you can meet your body's daily protein requirements whether you drink shakes or eat whole foods; however, protein powder contains fewer nutrients than whole foods. For that reason, shakes should not be your only food source. Whole food offers a much bigger nutritional punch. Liquid 'diets' are limited nutritionally and are not a sustainable way to eat. So, as I've outlined above, choose your protein powder based on your individualized needs and consider nutrient-timing to meet your dietary requirements and goals.

Limiting Alcohol (Plus my Approved Light Cocktails)

I know what you're thinking—do I have to give up alcohol to achieve my health and fitness goals?

I'm a true believer in not having to give up the things that you love; however, the word 'moderation' becomes key here. At seven calories per gram, alcohol has nearly as many calories as fat. So if your goal is fat loss, you can see how it's quite easy to blow your deficit. When you drink alcohol, your body's priority is to use alcohol (over carbohydrates and fat) for fuel. This is because the by-product of alcohol metabolism, acetate, is toxic. Only when your body has metabolized the alcohol will it revert to using carbs, so it takes longer to return to fat burn. Most alcohol is made from natural starch and sugar so it's a double-edged sword. Not to mention the toxicity factor and that after a few drinks your inhibitions weaken and your appetite is stimulated; you may find yourself eating whatever crosses your path!

That being said, having a glass of wine or a vodka soda isn't going to make or break your health and fitness goals. Heck, there are some health benefits to moderate intake of some alcohol.

These include lowering the risk of diabetes, gall and kidney stones, stroke, and cardiac arrest. Red wine also provides potent antioxidants and polyphenol (hello resveratrol!).

Let's take a closer look at which are the best types of alcohol to drink.

Which alcohols don't contain sugar?

There are a lot of pure alcohols that don't contain carbs; like spirits with high alcohol volume. Tequila, Gin, Vodka, Brandy, Whiskey, and Rum all have no carb content and can be seen as sugar-free. Due to the small volume you drink, they're also pretty low on calorie content; perfect for those on the hunt for sugar-free alcohol.

When it comes to spirits like these, it's the mixes you want to watch out for. Cocktails are high in sugar and calories, so I tend to choose soda water as my base and a squeeze of lemon or lime or fruit with fresh herbs. I always pack stevia drops or my monk fruit simple syrup (page 356). I use a few drops to add sweetness without the sugar. Sex it up a bit by adding some fresh basil or mint, and you've got my favorite, a sugar-free mojito. Check out the Mocktail Chapter to see all my favorites.

What about wine and beer?

Although you can't expect zero sugar in these alcoholic drinks, it's not all bad news.

It's nearly impossible to break down the nutritional value of each and every bottle of wine (and I don't think it's healthy to obsess over this anyway). Here are some general guidelines that can help you understand which is the best option.

Red wine

Thanks to the health benefits I mentioned above, red wine is one of the best choices for a lower sugar option. One serving, or a large (250 ml) glass of red wine, won't have a significant effect on your blood sugar or insulin levels and contains less than 2 grams of sugar (carbs); that's about 1/4 of a teaspoon of sugar. Of all wines, red has the lowest sugar content. Sweet wines will contain a bit more carbs.

White wine

White wine is where it gets a bit trickier. Dry white wine contains a lot less sugar than sweet white wine. For a 250 ml glass, you're looking at around 1.5 grams for the dry type and about 4 grams for the sweet kind. For a medium white? You guessed it: somewhere in the middle.

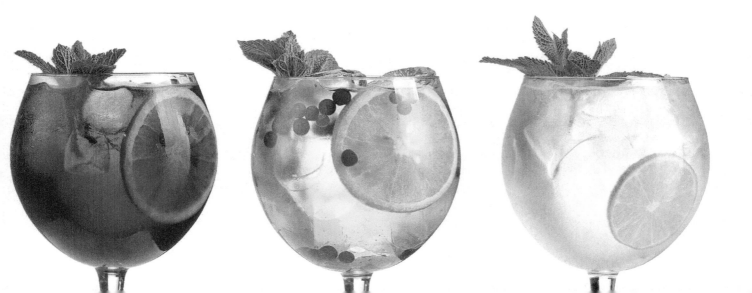

Beer

Beer has a spectrum of sugar content and, while it can be high in calories and carbohydrates, it tends to be relatively low in sugar content. That's because of the type of sugar molecules it contains. If you want the science talk, it contains oligosaccharides, which your body just can't digest. A 12 oz bottle of regular beer can contain up to 14 grams of carbs but zero grams of sugar. There are lower-carb beers, which contain around 5 g of carbs per bottle. Interestingly, lots of non-alcoholic beers have way more sugar—up to 29 grams. Read your labels!

Bubbles

A 100 ml glass of bubbly contains just 80 calories and a gram of sugar, well under a teaspoon. We raise our glasses to that news!

At the end of the day, weigh your fitness and health goals and decide what is most important to you. Whether cutting alcohol completely or staying within the moderate range, staying conscious about nutrition, adequate exercise, and knowing your drink limit is key. If you do choose to have a drink, be mindful of the type of alcohol and of the amount you consume—it's all about, you guessed it, balance!

The Facts on Salt and Hydration

Hydrations Tips

90% of new clients that apply to work with me are severely dehydrated. Water is the most underutilized tool when it comes to your health. From hydrating skin and helping with fat loss and performance, and preventing headaches to giving you an endless supply of energy and optimal gut health, simply drinking enough H_2O each day can pay off in a big way. Staying hydrated is one of the most important factors when it comes to a lean, healthy body. I always start my day with a large glass of water with some lemon and apple cider vinegar to help to alkalize my system and help improve insulin sensitivity. When you do this, it also helps your body carry more oxygen, so you're more energized!

It's important to not drink too much water during a meal because the liquid can dilute your stomach acids and cause your stomach to work harder when digesting foods.

If you're making an effort to reduce your body fat or overeat, use fluids to your advantage. Drink 2 cups of water before a meal to reduce your food intake - by as much as 13% according to some research. This is a great practice to adopt as over time it helps with fat loss.

But how much should you be drinking?

According to the Mayo Clinic, women should generally drink about 9 cups of fluids a day, while men should aim for 12. That's 72 ounces for us ladies, which is just over 2 liters. However, if you're active and live in a warm climate, you'll require more. Dehydration can produce several different side effects, from feeling a little lethargic to plummeting blood pressure. While everyone's sweat rate is different, it's safe to assume that for every 45 to 60 minutes of exercise you do, you'll need to drink a minimum of 40 ounces of H_2O—a number that will probably seem staggeringly high to some of you. Even if you don't have symptoms, you can still tell if you're falling short of your water needs. Just check the color of your pee. It should be a light straw color when you're staying properly hydrated! I always polish off my 1.5 L bottle of water during my workout and then I know I'm nearly at 50% of my daily water target. And, one of my greatest secrets is that I use one teaspoon of sea salt in my water bottle while I train. There's no better intra-workout drink than water and all those natural minerals!

I recommend around a gallon or 3.5 liters per day. If you're not anywhere near that, then slowly start adding more water every day, and you'll soon find that you're hitting that volume with ease. Aim to have about half of your planned water intake for the day consumed about halfway through your day. Making it a habit is key!

If you struggle to get in your water, there are loads of great water tracking apps. It can also help if you get a water bottle you love. Finally, when it comes to upping hydration, it doesn't just have to be plain H20. Teas and fruit-infused water are a great way to add some flavor to your water with some health benefits as well. Lemon water and infused waters are the best natural drinks for hormone balance as they improve your skin, control appetite, help to regulate blood sugar levels, and boost your overall immunity. Green tea and a matcha latte are two of my favorite green drinks with added hormone-balancing properties (without added sugar, of course!).

Spring, purified, mineral, alkaline artesian, tap water… What is the best water to drink?

This has always been a hot topic as we continue to see new brands of water hit the shelves and claim amazing health benefits. Here's the 4-1-1 on what these waters are and my personal opinion on which water to drink.

Spring water comes from an underground source and must be collected at the spring or through a borehole tapping the spring's source.

Purified water is water that has been highly treated, through distillation, deionization, or other suitable processes, to meet certain standards before being sold.

Mineral water is natural water that has a constant level and relative proportions of mineral and trace elements. It contains no less than 250 parts per million total of dissolved solids and minerals cannot be added to it.

Then there's artesian water, which is derived from a well that taps a specific layer of rock or sand.

You also might have seen alkaline water on store shelves (I know… so many to choose from). It has a higher pH level than tap water. A pH level is a measure of how acidic or basic water is. Seven is a neutral pH, higher pH levels are more alkaline or basic; lower pH levels are more acidic. I wouldn't pay more for this water as, in my opinion, there currently isn't enough evidence supporting the health claims made about alkaline water.

All of these waters are safe to drink. My first choice would be spring water, if it's from a quality spring, as this water will have all the natural minerals that are removed during the purification process with filtered water. You can also add your minerals back into your water with a supplement or drops, which can be easily found online.

When it comes to drinking tap water in countries where it's safe to do so, I would always use a water filtration system. Tap water has been found to be polluted all across the U.S., containing endocrine-disrupting chemicals (not good for our hormones), chlorine, and even arsenic. Even though these limits are considered 'safe,' I filter my water if drinking from a tap source. There are some great, inexpensive options available like carbon filtering and, if you have a slightly larger budget, reverse osmosis. Do your research and choose a reputable brand with lab reports.

For me, the bottom line is that drinking enough water daily is far more important than the type of water you drink. Get that water in!

Salt

Don't kick the salt! You may have heard that you need to cut out salt, but salt is an important nutrient for the human body. Your body uses salt to keep electrolytes in balance and maintain healthy blood pressure. It's also essential for nerve, hormone, and muscle function. Not only that but also salt is arguably one of the world's most important cooking ingredients. Without it, most meals would taste bland and unappealing—however, a pinch goes a long way. One meal out in a restaurant could easily push you over the recommended daily sodium limit of 1500 mg per day. When eating a diet of mostly unprocessed, whole foods, I recommend a dash of salt on all your meals. Avoid regular table salt as it's highly refined and choose a salt with a higher mineral content that includes iodine (which supports the thyroid gland) such as Himalayan pink salt, kosher salt, sea salt, or Celtic salt.

Ways to Balance Your Hormones With the Food on Your Plate

When your hormones are balanced you'll achieve your health and fitness goals much easier period. Hormones have a huge (and often under emphasized) impact on our overall health and well-being as they affect everything from our menstrual cycles to health issues such as PCOS, Thyroid, Infertility, PMS, and Endometriosis. While these symptoms may be the 'normal' experience for many women, they don't have to be your normal! Perimenopause and menopause don't have to be the worst times of our lives. Nutrition can be a powerful tool when addressing hormone imbalance. When hormones are in harmony, like a symphony, you feel like a superhuman—at any age. Although more research is needed in this area, we already know so much about how the food you eat can support optimal hormone health. Through my 1x1 coaching, I've been able to help many women upregulate their metabolism and optimize their hormones by upgrading lifestyle factors, with the major one being what's on the end of their fork. I'm not going to deep dive into this (this topic could be an entire book by itself!), but I'm going to share a brief overview of how you can start to help your hormones through nutrition.

Support Your Thyroid By Eating These Foods:

Seafood- excellent food choice to help balance your thyroid. Seafood has selenium and iodine, which are both great vitamins for hormones.

Mustard Greens- high in tyrosine

Brazil Nuts- high in selenium

Sea Vegetables (dulce, nori and wakame are my favorites)- high in iodine

Pumpkin Seeds- a great source of zinc and tyrosine. Eat a handful of pumpkin seeds a day to increase your levels.

Spinach (Buy Organic)- this includes magnesium, iron, and tyrosine, which are needed for optimal thyroid function.

Consuming a balance of both warm and cold foods is key. Avoid excessive cold, raw, and 'damp' foods. Try to eat more grilled or baked foods that are warm in temperature and add warming spices.

Here are a couple examples of foods to add to your diet:

Organic Chicken with the skin on - This includes fat-soluble vitamins. Consume a blend of chicken with the skin on and off.

Sweet Potatoes- includes vitamin A which can help the thyroid hormone within your body's cells.

Oranges- This fruit contains vitamin C, which is excellent to pair with iron rich food since vitamin C can help the absorption of iron.

Bone Broth- includes magnesium and vitamin A which is vital for thyroid health. It can also help gut health, which can affect the majority of our bodily processes-especially hormones.

Eat more small and frequent meals with enough protein to ensure blood sugar regulation. This can help reduce excess cortisol production and regulate adrenal activity.

Regulate Blood Sugar By Including These Foods (to help insulin imbalance):

Increase High Fiber Foods - These can consist of flaxseed, black beans, & chia seeds. Adding some flax or chia seeds over a salad or in yogurt is a great way to easily add extra fiber to your diet.

Include whole, unprocessed foods.

These are excellent herbs to stabilize blood sugar:

**Cinnamon • Bitter Melon • Licorice • Barberry
Ashwagandha • Fenugreek • Gymnema**

Incorporate These Foods To Balance Estrogen Levels:

High Fiber Foods- These help your good gut bacteria and help move that extra estrogen out. Simply adding some chia seeds to a smoothie or on top of a salad is an easy way to incorporate some fiber. You can also add flax seeds to recipes as well. Most of my recipes have you covered!

Broccoli- One of my favorite foods to balance hormones! Broccoli is packed with anti-cancer properties and has excellent fiber content. Sauteing some up with rice and onions and other veggies is an easy way to add these to your meals.

Herbal Powders that are great for Female Hormones are:	Add Loose Herbal Teas that include:
Maca Licorice Ginger Ashwagandha Rhodiola Dioscorea Angelica S. Eleutherococcus	Motherwort Oat straw Lemon balm Red Clover Nettles Raspberry leaf Ginger

Foods & Minerals That Can Balance Testosterone Levels

Zinc is a vital mineral that can help balance out testosterone levels.

Seeds- include more seeds like pumpkin, hemp or sesame seeds

Legumes- chickpeas, beans, and lentils are a great source of zinc.

Nuts- pine nuts, cashews and almonds can all be a great grab and go snack to help your levels.

Include These Foods in Your Diet to Aid Progesterone Levels:

Zinc is mostly known to help with balancing testosterone, as mentioned above. However, zinc plays a critical role in progesterone levels too. Eat foods that are high in zinc, like those listed under the testosterone section above.

Also, add Vitamin B6 rich foods to your diet as well. Vitamin B6 is essential in progesterone metabolism. Certain medications, like the birth control pill, can deplete your progesterone levels. You may benefit from incorporating foods like chickpeas, organic chicken, and wild salmon into your diet.

Additional Ways to Help Your Hormones Reset

Follow a consistent sleep/bedtime routine. Without quality sleep, your insulin and cortisol will suffer.

Control your stress to keep cortisol levels healthy by practicing mindfulness, breathing techniques, meditation, yoga, and mind/ body practices.

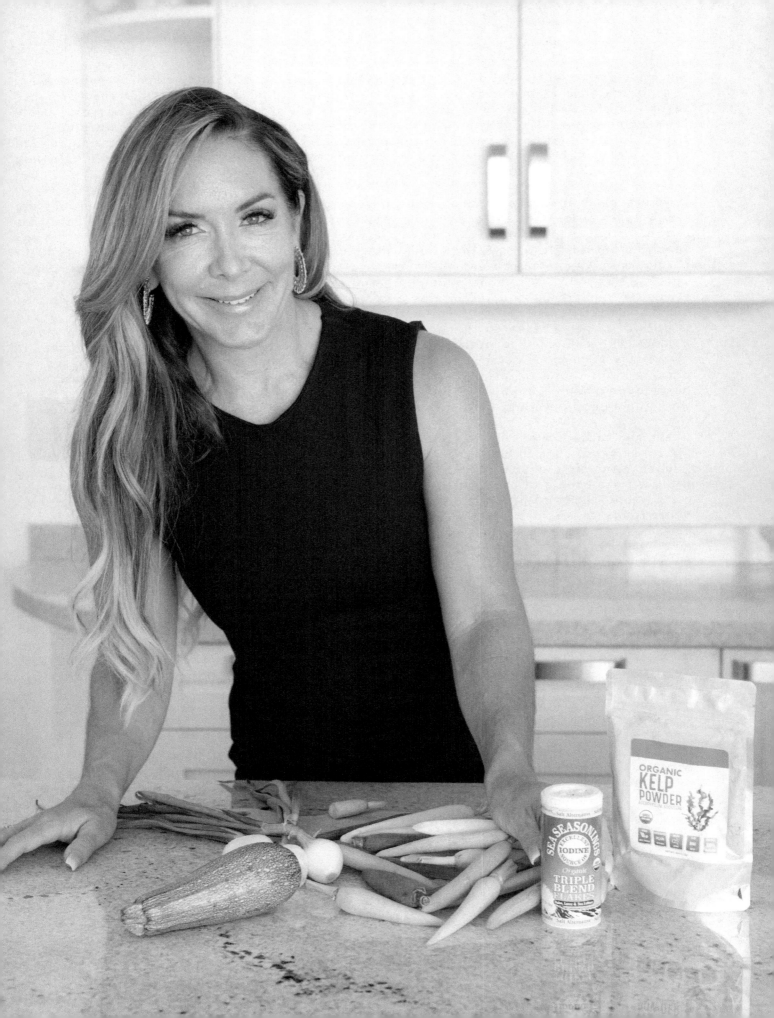

Get moving. Get your sweat on, girl! Exercise has a powerful effect on balancing, suppressing, and increasing certain hormones. Excess estrogen, insulin, and cortisol are the hormones responsible for weight gain, while HGH, testosterone, and progesterone are the ones responsible for keeping us lean. I'm not going to dive too deeply into this here, but you want to design a fitness routine that has some HIIT (High-Intensity Interval Training), strength training (even body weight and Pilates), and stretching or yoga. Always listen to how your body is feeling when it comes to daily movement.

If you're perimenopausal or menopausal, you may want to try some intermittent fasting (12-16 hours of fasting) and see how you feel. Intermittent Fasting is an eating pattern that alternates between periods of eating and fasting. Intermittent fasting could take place in any specified period, although 8/16 (8 hours in which you can eat, 16 hours of fasting) and 10/14 (10 hours in which you can eat, 14 hours of fasting) are the two most common approaches. There are actually various methods of intermittent fasting, and people will prefer different styles, so don't be afraid to try this and see if it's a dietary lifestyle that suits you. Of course, a Nutritionist can help you with a personalized plan and to avoid setbacks. There is a lot of positive research that suggests intermittent fasting may help improve hormonal balance. This can enhance metabolism and sleep, leave us feeling more energized and help us effectively burn more calories. As women age into perimenopausal/menopausal years, we become more prone to insulin resistance (Insulin resistance is a state in which your body has enough insulin available to handle your blood glucose levels and chooses not to). Fasting would be a good option to help improve insulin resistance.

I have had success with some fasting in my forties. I apply fasting when my body feels for it. I use my hunger cues to guide me. If I'm not feeling hungry, then I'll implement a fast. When I do it, I either fast weekly 24 hours or fast intermittently for 16 hours with an 8 hour feeding window for a couple of days per week, and love the 'lighter' feeling I have afterward as well as the opportunity to practice discipline. My focus always remains on balance and nutrient-dense foods (my recipes!), just with a reduced feeding window. Fasting doesn't work for me as an exclusive dietary lifestyle—because I love food too much! And I exercise early in the morning most days, and I perform and recover best with food around my workouts. I also guide my clients with an individualized approach to fasting if we determine it's an appropriate dietary lifestyle for them. I would not try fasting if your relationship with food still needs improvement, you experience extreme hunger that causes you to binge eat, you feel dizzy, or you have diabetes (especially if you take medication to lower blood sugar). If you want to try intermittent fasting, start slowly, by extending the time between your dinner and breakfast (cut the late-night snacking!), and see how you feel. Try it again in a couple of days and reassess again. The more you do it the easier it should become. Always listen to your body. Don't feel great? Then there's no reason to continue. Always remember, as women, different seasons of our life call for different lifestyles. What works for you at one moment might not work for you at another and it's important to never get stuck in a style of eating that doesn't serve you. That's when it becomes a diet.

If you're concerned that you have a hormone imbalance, it's important to have your hormones checked through blood tests. I require hormone blood tests from my clients as part of my onboarding process and work closely with their physicians that specialize in women's health to identify any imbalances. HRT (hormone replacement therapy) should never be used before optimal nutrition and healthy lifestyle practices are in place. We should always start with the foundation and, if HRT is required then take those next steps.

When it comes to balancing hormones, I've learned it's essential to consider hormone production, regulation, and elimination. Any one of these problems can cause hormone imbalances. So, adding or taking hormones doesn't necessarily fix the problem. We must

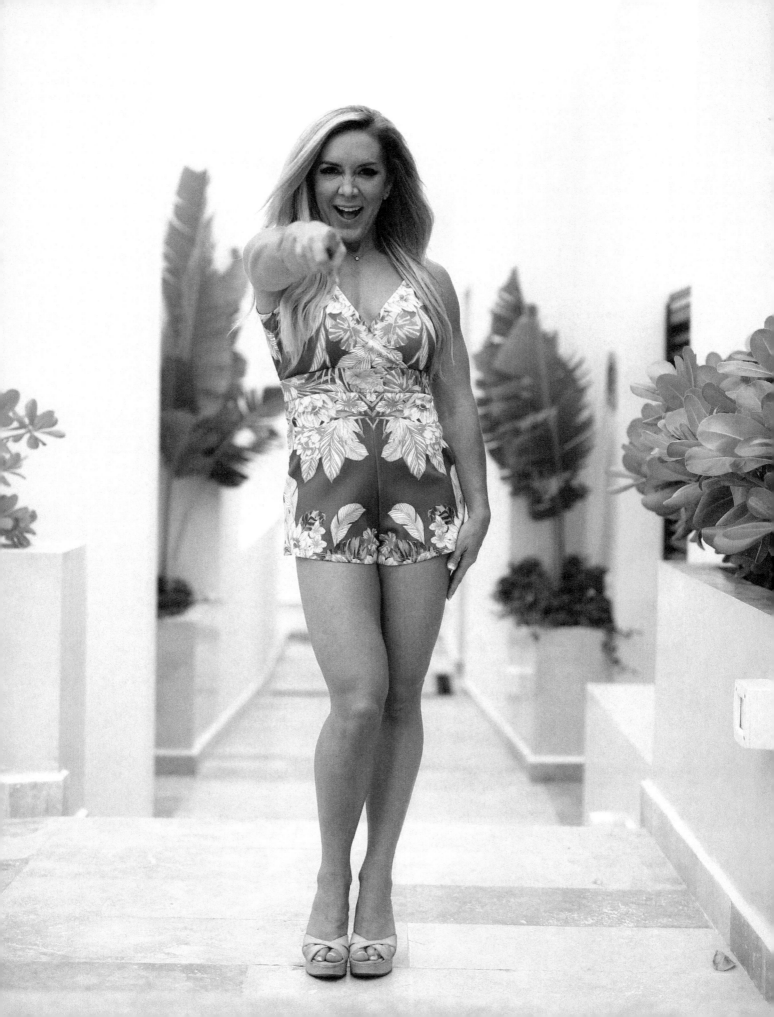

consider regulation, so even if you have an optimal amount, your body might not be able to use it correctly. Once you have a truly healthy hormone balance, you'll feel better all around. You'll have improved body composition, stronger bones, reduced PMS, better sleep, a healthy stress response, a regular menstrual cycle or improved menopause symptoms, and increased energy and mood. This will be a lifestyle change. It's not going to be fixed overnight, so be patient and consistent. Pick a couple of easy steps from these tips and get started!

Should I take Supplements?

I'm often asked if we can obtain all of our nutrients from food. This would make sense if we were eating a completely clean diet, however, in today's world, due to depleted soils, high stress, processed foods, and environmental toxins, we often fall short nutrient wise. This is why I use some supplements as an 'insurance policy' to fill in the nutritional gaps with some vitamins and minerals in addition to using them for repair and healing.

When chosing to take a supplement or not I always take a 'food first' approach. You can't out supplement a bad diet. If you focus on eating the rainbow daily you'll be off to a great start and may or may not feel the need to add supplements to your diet. We all have a different biology, needs, budgets and lifestyles, which should all be considered.

Some of my top 10 supplements for health and wellness are:

---

1) Multi-vitamin
2) Broad spectrum probiotic
3) Omega 3
4) Magnesium
5) Vitamin K2/D3
6) Ashwaghanda
7) CoQ10
8) Berberine
9) Methyl B-12
10) Electrolytes

I take some of these occasionally or daily, depending on my needs at that time. For instance, when I travel I always take my supplements as I know I won't be eating as optimally as when I'm at home. Chose to take a supplement wisely and only if you feel your body requires it. Also, always purcahse high quality supplements that do not contain fillers, are free of toxins and are made in a facility with good manufacturing standards.

Putting it all Together and Keeping it Together

Almost anyone can get on the healthy bandwagon for a week or two. The true challenge lies in making this a lifestyle. I know you're busy, but your health is the single best investment you can ever make. You don't have time to be sick or feel like garbage, so invest your time wisely, superstar!
Staying dedicated to your nutrition isn't just about your food. Yes, this information and recipes are life-changing, but they're just one part of an interconnected, healthy lifestyle. Now I know this book isn't about fitness, sleep, meditation, journaling, self-care, or stress management but it wouldn't be complete without mentioning the importance of designing and maintaining a winning wellness routine on the quest to becoming your best self. Improving one area of your life inspires you to improve others. Plus you'll generate momentum when you make your other soul-nourishing activities a priority. If you're not sweating daily, this is a habit you'll

want to adopt. Whether that's gentle yoga, hitting the weights, or pushing yourself to the maximum intensity with a HIIT cardio session, moving daily is going to pay off dividends. Exercise is an amazing mood-booster and is great for our health, not to mention a self-confidence booster. I suggest more strength training versus cardio as we age because it helps to maintain strong bones and joints, supports hormones, improves metabolism and insulin sensitivity, and can make incredible improvements in your body composition (less fat and more muscle). Sleep and stress management are two other pillars of wellness that must be a top priority to see and feel results. Take the time to look at your life and start to design a wellness routine that nourishes what you need most in your life. If you're not getting optimal sleep you're going to find it nearly impossible to stay on track with healthy eating as you'll be craving all things full of sugar! Finding effective ways to manage your stress will help manage your cortisol levels, which is imperative for a healthy, happy body. Drip in moments of self-care to fill up your cup. Some of my favorites are going for a walk in the sunshine, going to the beach to connect with nature, cuddles from Zuri, getting a massage, having a date night with Marcelo, video calls with my family and friends, reading a book, meditating or having a bath. Your nutrition is fueling your body, which keeps you going, but your soul is fueled by love and joy. I recommend multiple servings of laughs daily!

Remember, motivation is the outcome of getting started. You won't always feel motivated, and every day won't always be an awesome day, but when you commit yourself to show up as your highest self every day, I promise you it's going to become easier. You're going to start feeling better and you're going to start looking better. Start slowly, stay consistent, and enjoy this journey!

It's time to take the next step. Are you ready to get cooking?! Let's get in the kitchen!

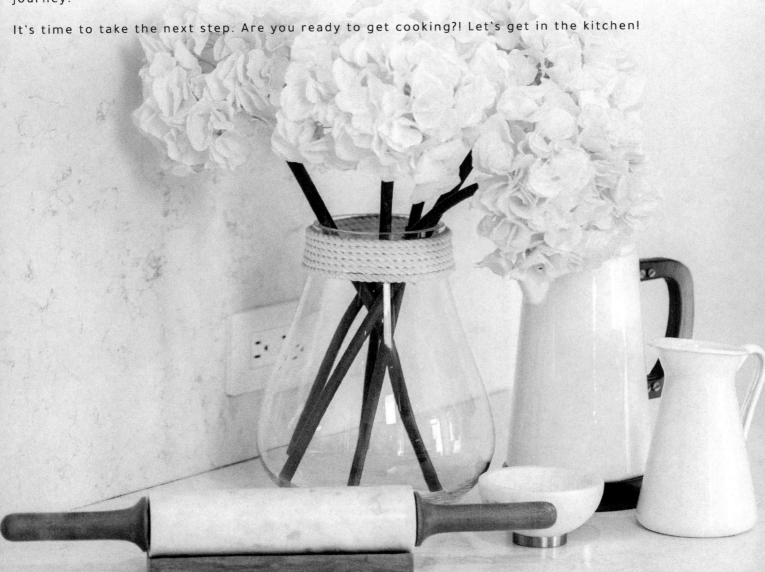

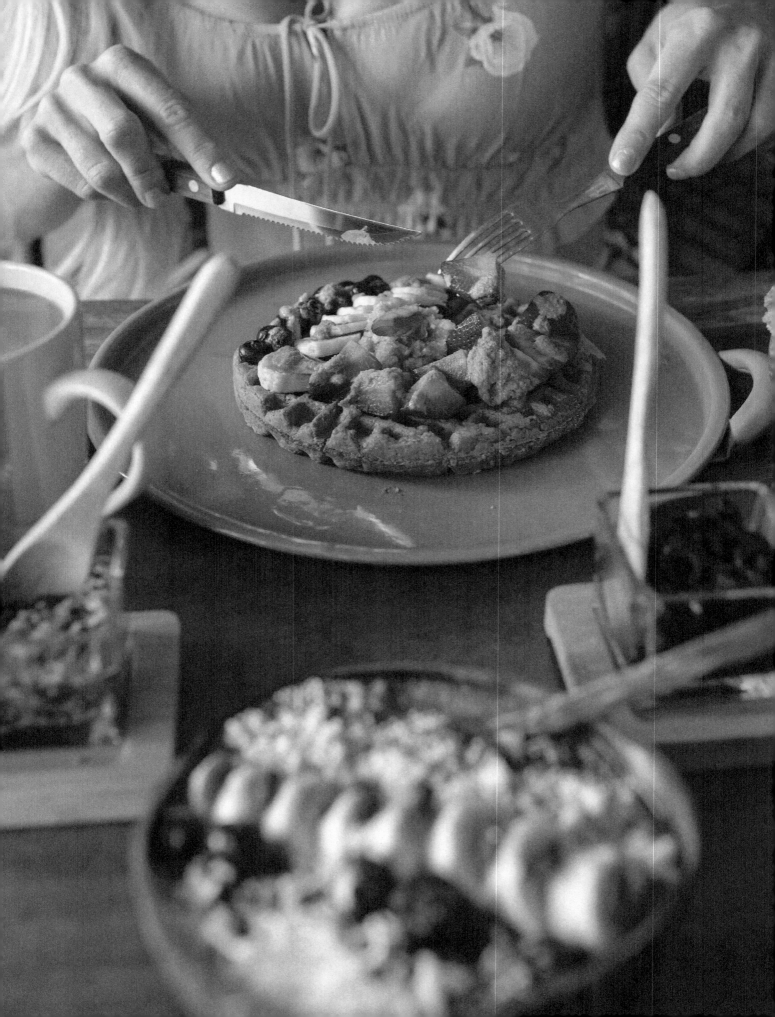

RECIPES TO THRIVE

Contents

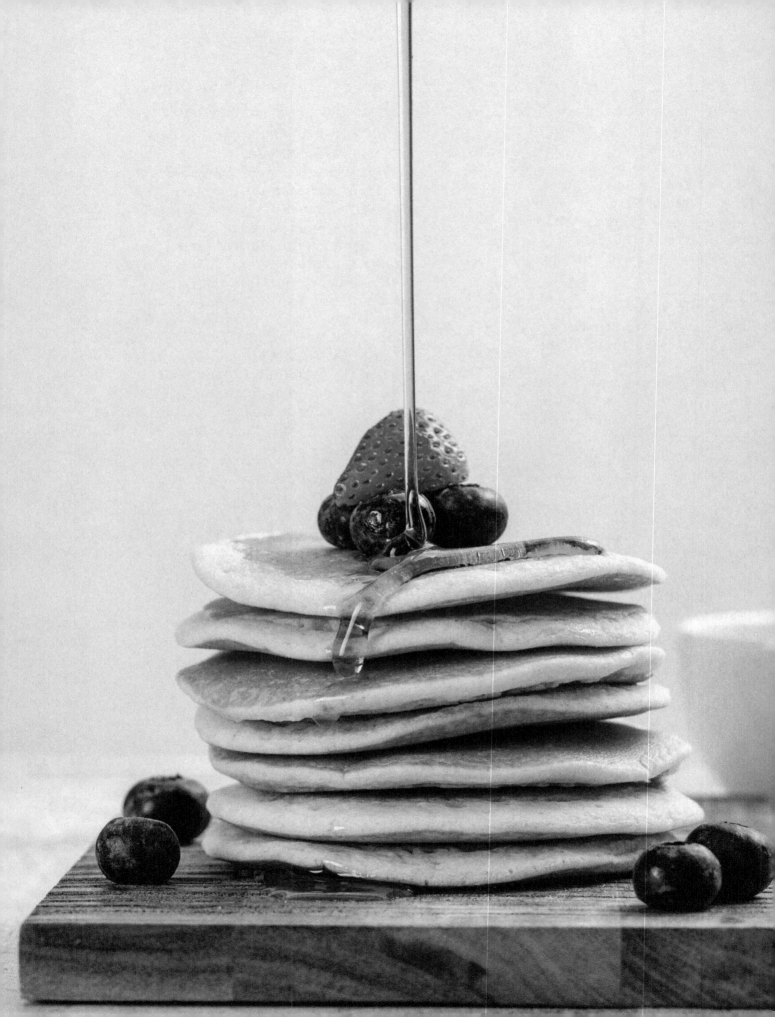

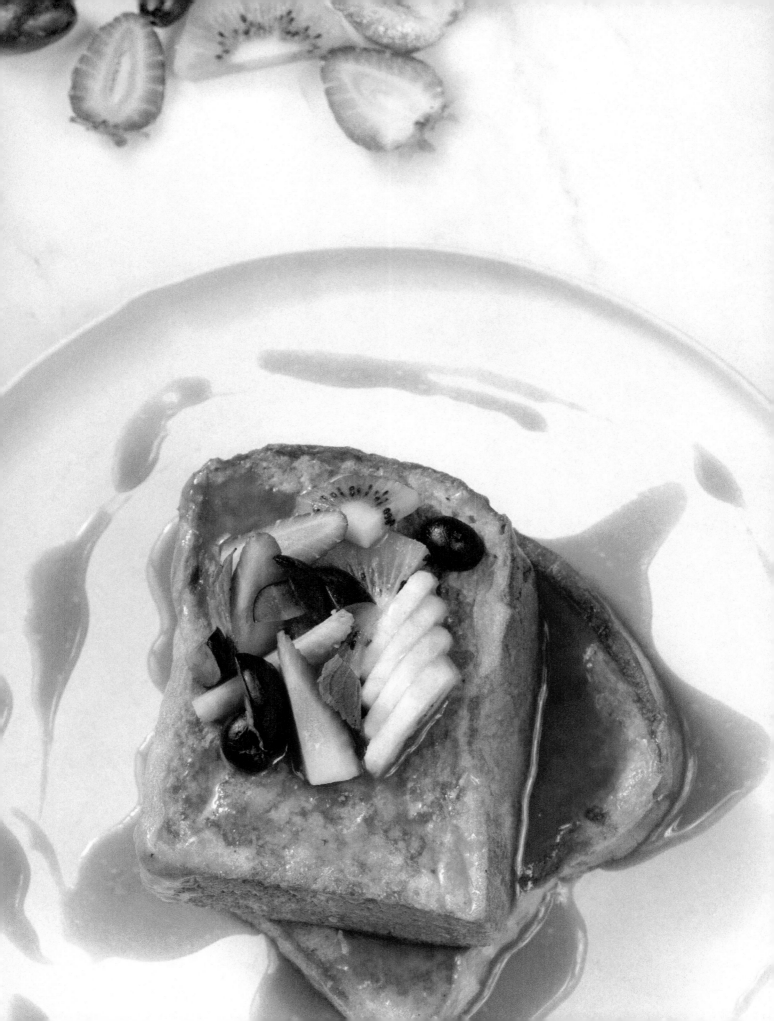

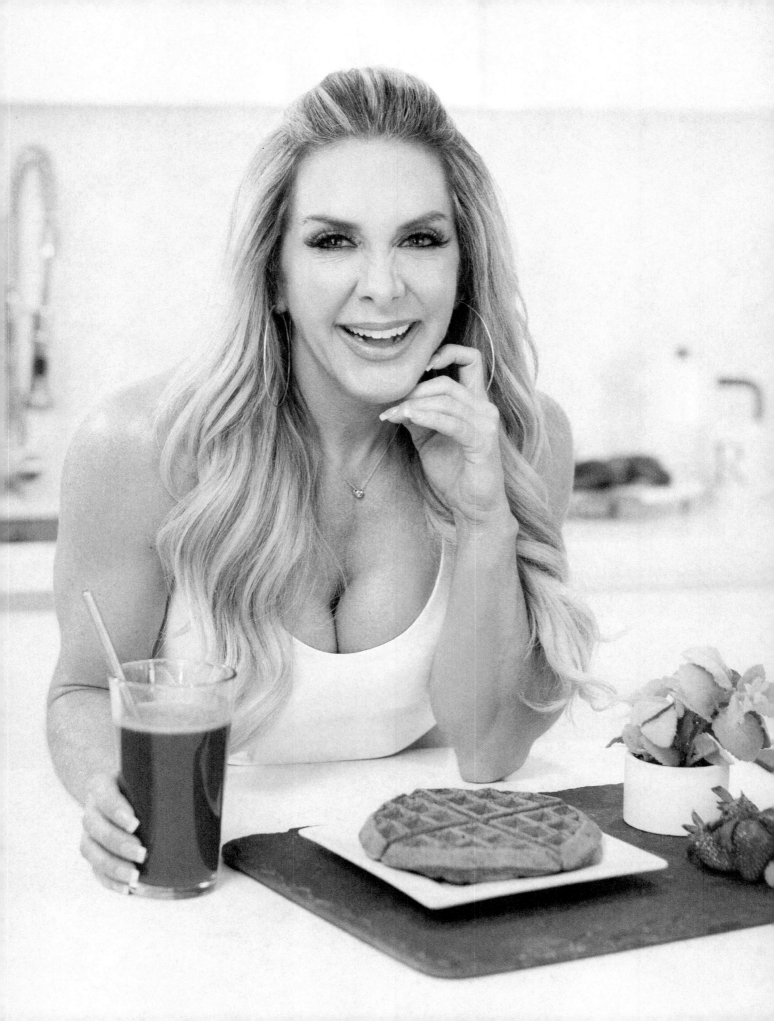

Hulk Waffles

Eating your veggies for breakfast has never been so easy or tasted so good!
My signature waffles are going to WOW you and your family. Loaded with nutrition,
flavor and fiber - these are the waffles you can feel good about eating.
They also make a great portable snack and your kids will love them!
This is my go-to airplane meal and one of my favorite meals to send to school with Zuri.

Ingredients

2.............. whole egg

1 cup .... egg whites

1 cup .... oatmeal or oat flour

2 tsp......... flax seed

2 tsp......... chia seed

2 tsp......... coconut oil

2 cup .... spinach

2/3 .... large, banana

Preparation

1. Combine all of the ingredients in a blender until smooth.

2. Meanwhile, heat your waffle iron and use a light amount of coconut oil to grease the pan and pour in waffle mixture. Once mixture starts to form and bubbles appear on top flip the waffle and cook on the other side or a further 1 minute.

3. Tastes delicious topped with half a cup of berries, sugar free syrup and my protein whip cream!

Nutrition Facts
Servings: **2**
Calories Per Serving: **380**
Macros:
Protein: 23g
Total Carbs: 37.5g
Fat: 15.5g

RyFit Tip:
Add a 1/4 cup of protein powder to boost protein without ruining the consistency or flavor.

Blueberry Maple Turkey Breakfast Patties

If you're someone who likes meat for breakfast this is a healthy twist on the preservative-laden classic patties you'll find in stores and restaurants. These sweet & savory paleo blueberry maple turkey sausage breakfast patties with delicious spices and juicy blueberries hit the spot for breakfast or a satisfying protein option anytime. Serve these yummy patties with fresh fruit and eggs for the ultimate, high-protein low carb breakfast!
Super easy to make once you have all the ingredients on hand.

Ingredients

1 lb........... 93% lean ground turkey (do not use extra lean)

2............. garlic cloves, finely minced

1 tbsp .... sugar free maple syrup

1 tbsp .... fresh chopped sage (about 4 medium sage leaves)

1/2 tsp ...... thyme, dried

1/2 tsp ...... cumin, ground

1/2 tbsp..... ginger, ground

1/4 tbsp..... allspice

1/4 tbsp..... cayenne pepper

1/2 tsp ...... salt

1/2 tsp ...... pepper

1/3 cup...... blueberries, fresh or frozenc

Preparation

1. Place all ingredients besides the blueberries and oil in a large bowl and use your hands to mix until well combined. Add in blueberries and gently incorporate them into the meat. Form into 8 even sized patties, about 1/3 inch thick. Make sure the blueberries are tucked into the meat or they may pop out upon cooking.

2. Add 1 teaspoon coconut oil to a nonstick skillet and place over medium heat. Add turkey patties and cook for about 5 minutes then flip and cook for another 4-5 minutes or until fully cooked.

Nutrition Facts
Servings: **4**
Calories Per Serving: **194**
Macros:
Protein: 21.5g
Total Carbs: 7.8g (2g Fiber)
Fat: 3g

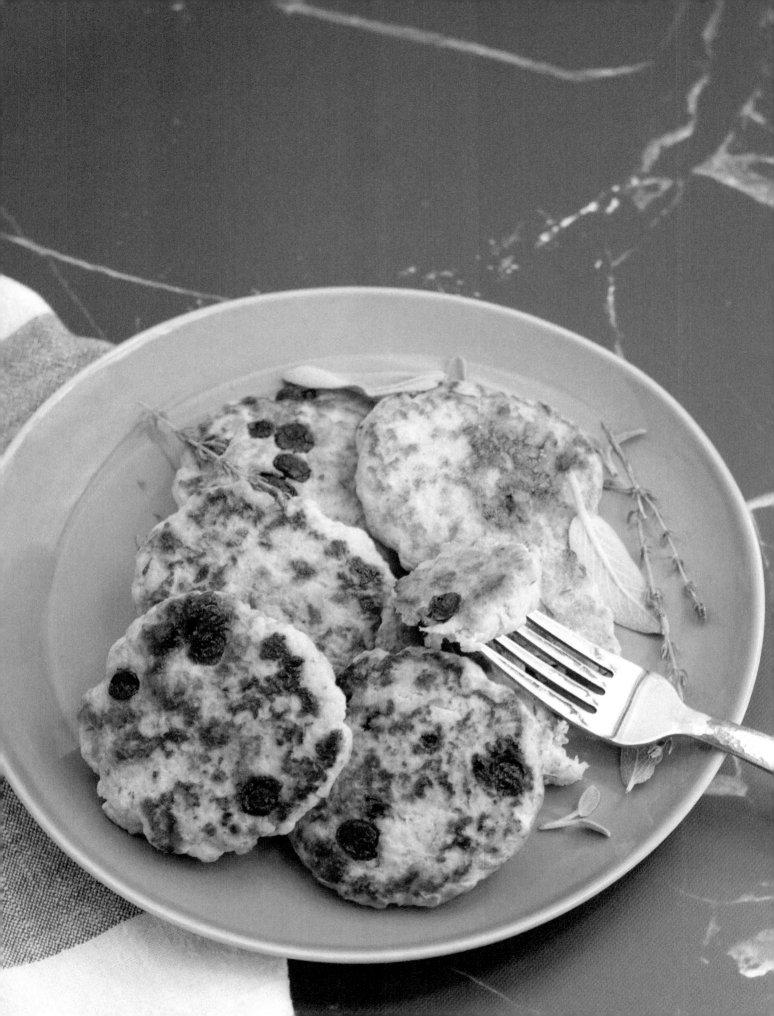

Fit Breakfast Toast

My healthy twist on a traditional breakfast sandwich. This satisfying breakfast hits the spot when you're feeling for a savory meal versus a sweet one!

Ingredients

1 . . . . whole egg

3 . . . . egg whites

1 cup . . . . spinach

1 strip . . . . turkey bacon or 1 extra egg white

1 tsp . . . . avocado

1 . . . . piece Ezekiel sprouted grain
or sourdough bread

1/2 . . . . tomato, medium

2 tbsp . . . . onion, diced

Preparation

In a nonstick pan combine all eggs and cook sunny side up. Sauté spinach for about 1 minute, then pan fry the turkey bacon. Toast the Ezekiel bread and when bread is warm, spread the avocado on first then add spinach, turkey bacon and cooked eggs. Add another piece of bread on top to make a breakfast sandwich.

Nutrition Facts

Servings: **1**

Calories Per Serving: **290**

Macros:

Protein: 23g

Total Carbs: 22g

Fat: 12g

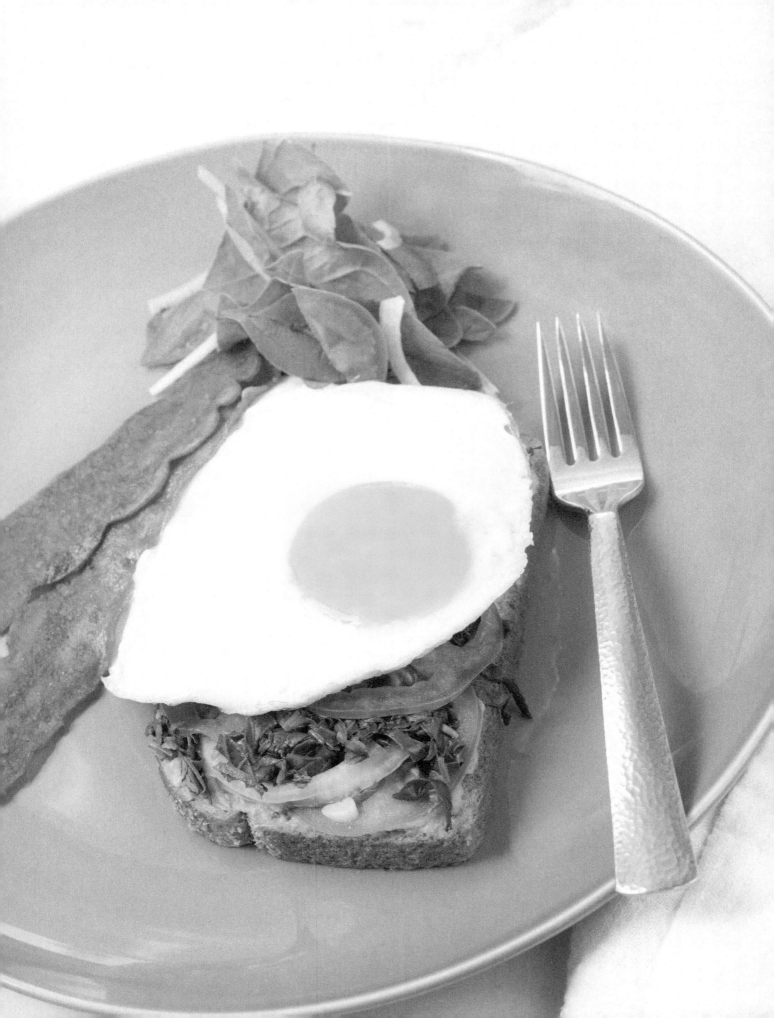

Protein Crepes

Say hello to a satisfying, high-protein snack...perfect for a light breakfast or a late night snack to curb hunger and promote quality sleep - get in my belly!

Crepe Ingredients

1/8 cup ...... oat flour

1 tbsp .... coconut flour

1/2 cup ..... protein powder

1 .... whole egg

3 .... egg whites

1 tsp .... cinnamon

1/4 cup ..... unsweetened dairy free milk

Filling Ingredients

2 tbsp .... protein whip cream

1/2 cup ...... fruit of choice

Optional fillings and toppings:

nut butter, cacao nibs, nuts, seeds

Preparation

1. In a medium bowl hand mix all ingredients together with a whisk until the batter is smooth.

2. Pour into a large nonstick pan or lightly sprayed, warm frying pan on medium heat. It's important to use a large frying pan so you have a thin consistency. You'll want to pour a thin amount of batter to create the perfect crepe consistency.

3. Flip carefully in 1-2 minutes when the batter bubbles.

4. Fill them with your filling of choice, roll into a crepe and add your toppings.

Nutrition Facts

Servings: **2**

Calories Per Serving: **144**

Macros:
Protein: 15.5g
Total Carbs: 11g (3.5g Fiber)
Fat: 4g

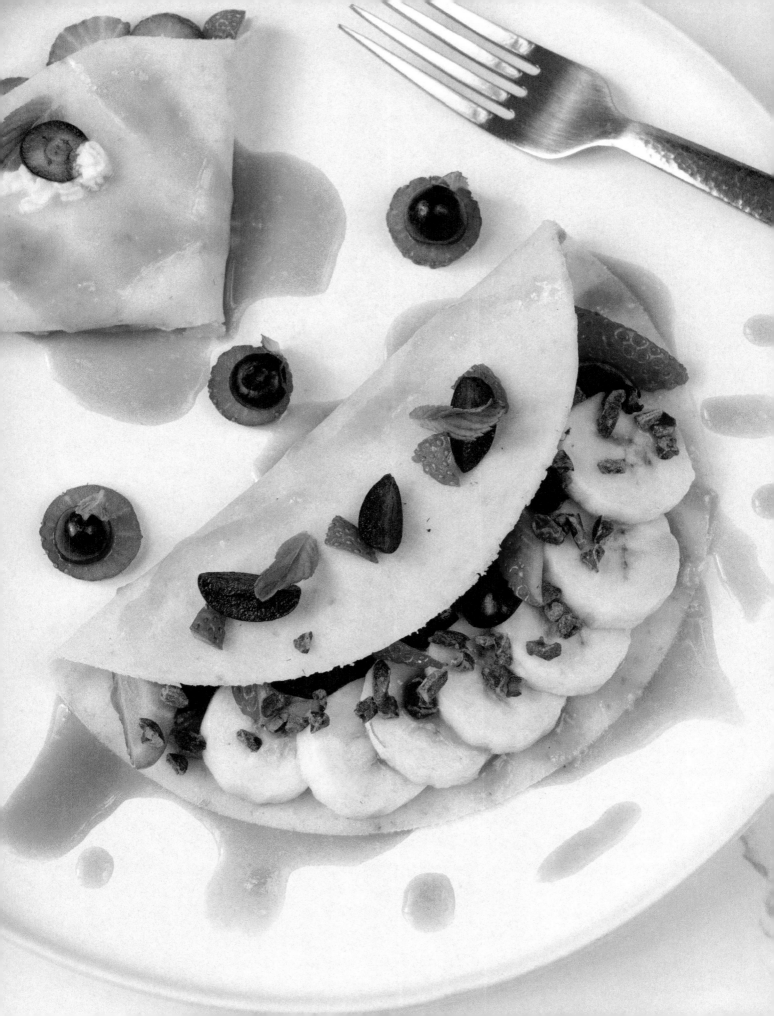

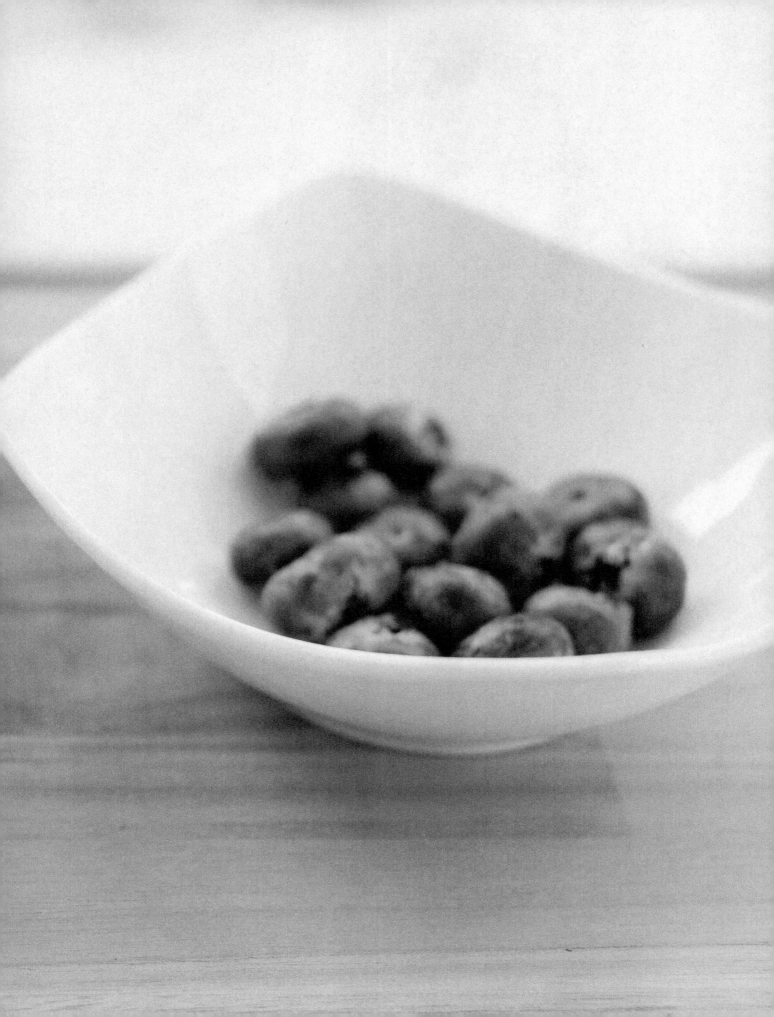

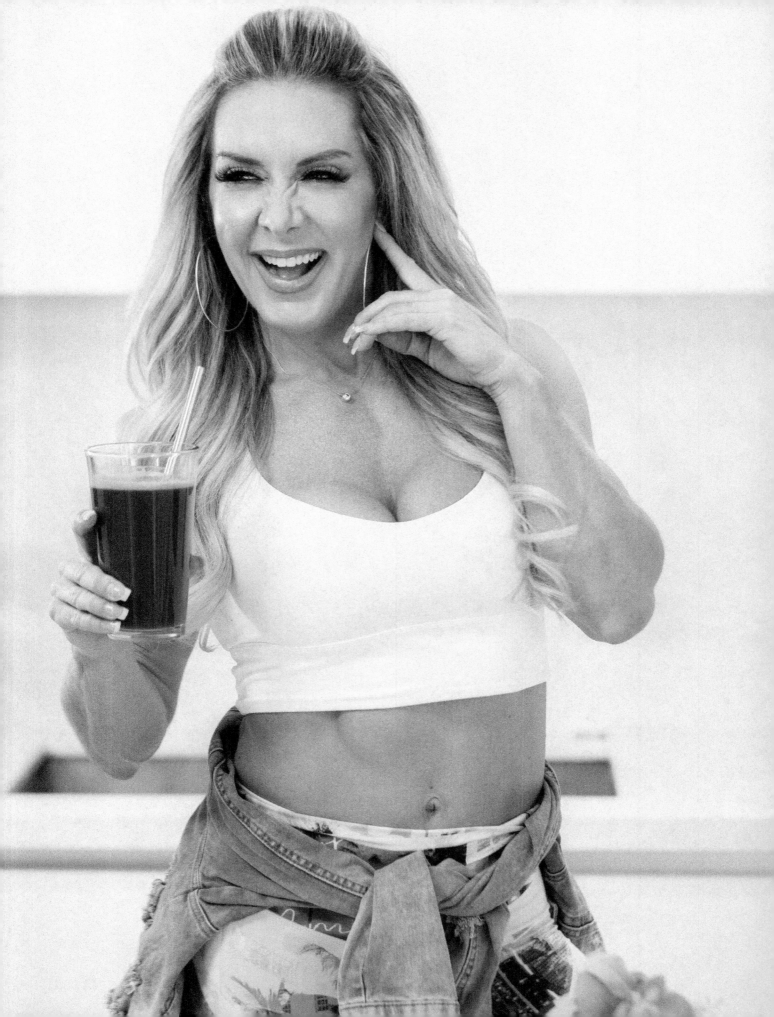

FRESH JUICES

Mom said it best. Eat your vegetables

With the pace of modern life the struggle is REAL when it comes to getting in enough fresh fruits and vegetables daily. Juicing provides a solution as a simple way to meet your daily requirements, increase your vitality and reap all the health benefits that freshly juiced produce has to offer. Bring on reduced rates of heart disease, high blood pressure, inflammation and some cancers and say hello to better energy, immunity and all of the powerful, preventative health benefits found in the colorful phytonutrients (your personal bodyguards against free radicals and diseases!) in plant foods.

Juicing is a healthy habit we're obsessed with in our home - we juice in the morning with a cold press juicer and drink it with breakfast. My simple recipes are 100-125 calories per serving with low sugar content. I don't promote juicing as meal replacements but rather as a 'nutritional boost' to compliment your meal. I love the clean flood of energy and mental focus I feel from it and it helps curb my cravings for sugar. More nutrition means we'll feel less prone to sugar cravings, more energized and sharper. This is turn helps us make smarter choices on repeat!

My guidelines on combining fruits and veggies are to chose 75% vegetables and 25% fruit for some sweetness while keeping the sugar low to avoid overly raising blood sugar levels. I love a celery or cucumber base and somedays I just end up juicing whatever veggies are nearly spoiled to avoid waste. Add a bit of fruit and lemon or ginger and you're set - it doesn't have to be fancy to be effective! These are my top simple juice recipes to supercharge your health and energize your day.

Brighten & Lighten

Servings: **2**

Ingredients:

1	Granny Smith apple, large
1 cup	spinach, tightly packed
1	cucumber, small
2	leaves Swiss chard
2	celery, stalks
1/4 cup......	cilantro leaves and stems
1/4	lemon, peeled

Cool as a Cucumber

Servings: **2**

Ingredients:

2 cups	green cabbage
2 cups	arugula
1	cucumber, smalll
2	celery, stalks
2	Granny Smith apples
1 inch........	ginger, peeled

Herbal Elixir

Servings: **2**

Ingredients:

1	cucumber, large
1 3/4 cup....	pineapple (frozen is ok)
1/4 cup......	basil leaves and stems
1/4 cup......	cilantro or parsley leaves and stems
1/4 cup......	mint leaves, tightly packed
1 inch........	ginger, peeled
4	kale, stalks

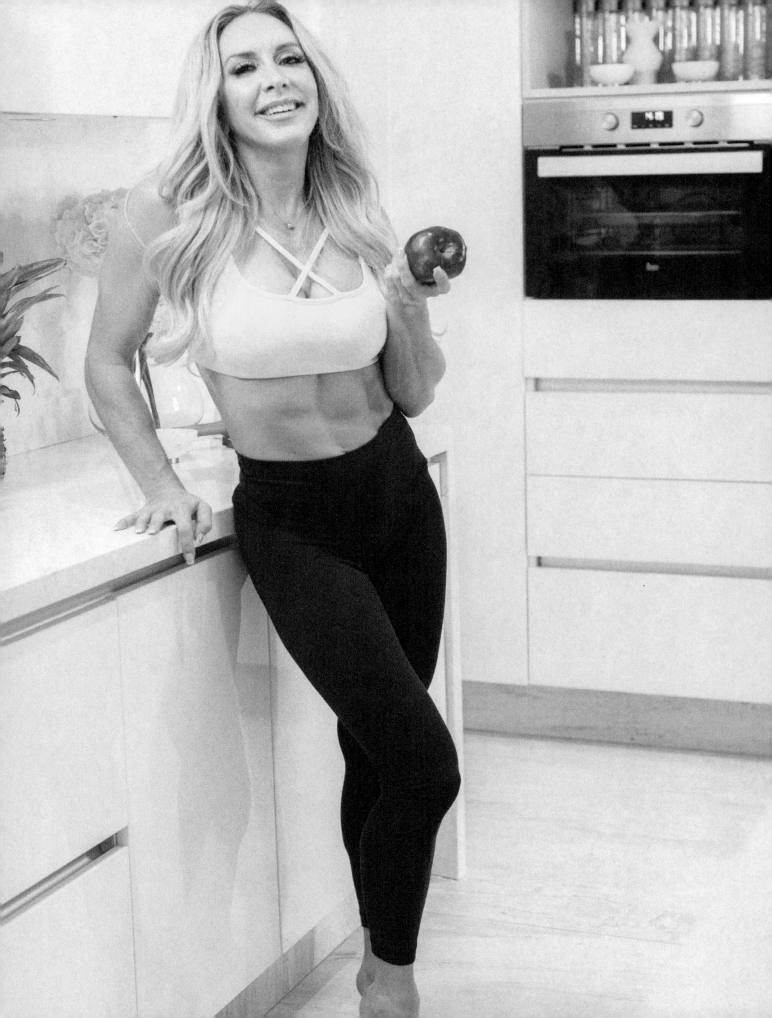

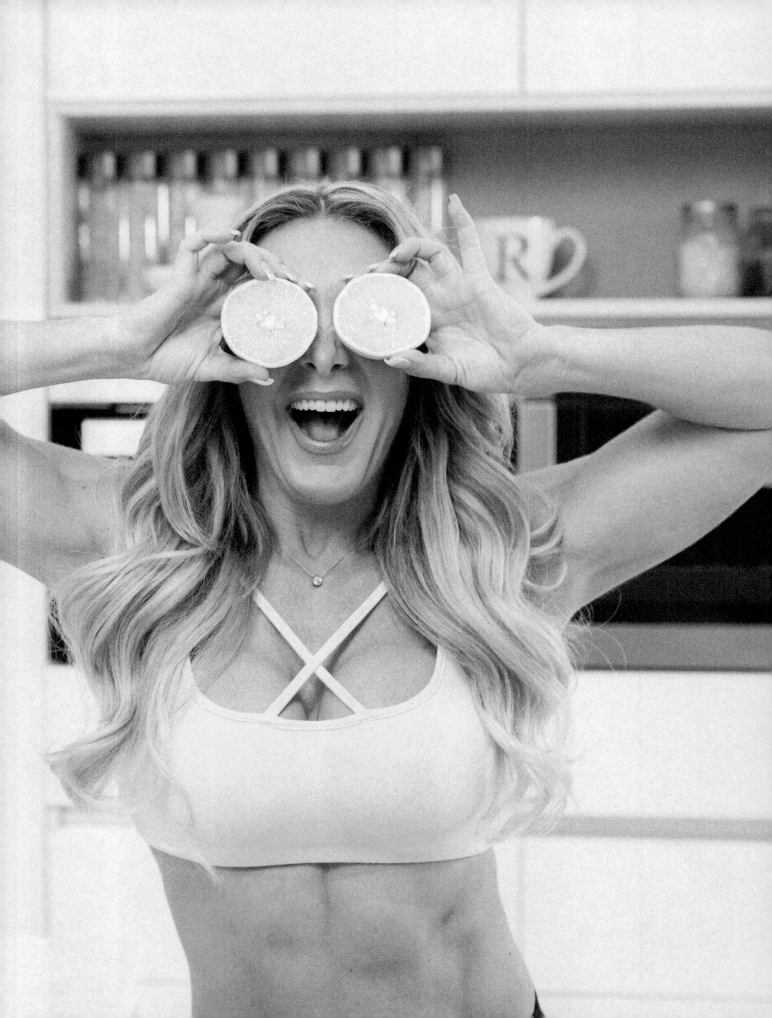

Liver Love

Servings: **2**

Ingredients:

4 .... carrots, medium
1 .... beet, medium
1 .... naval orange, medium, peeled
1 .... red bell pepper, seeds and stem removed
2 .... celery, stalks
1/4-1 inch ... ginger, peeled

Simple Greens & Carrot

Servings: **2**

Ingredients:

1 .... carrots, medium
1 .... cucumber, medium
1 .... celery, large stalk
1/4 cup ...... parsley leaves and stems
2 .... granny smith apples
1/2 .... head romaine lettuce, leaves only (8-10 leaves)

Vitamin C Bomb

Servings: **2**

Ingredients:

1 .... cucumber, medium
4 .... celery, stalks
2 .... small apples, cored and seeded
1 1/2 cup .... red cabbage
1/4 cup ...... mint leaves, tightly packed
1 inch .... ginger, peeled

155

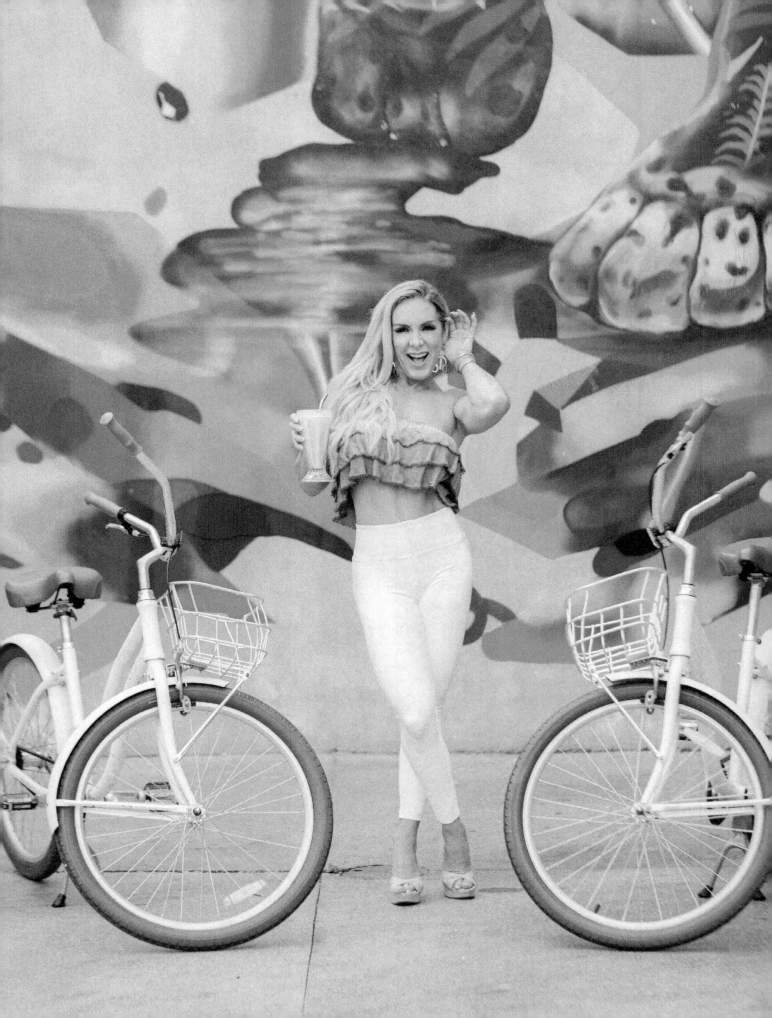

SNACKS AND PROTEIN SHAKES

Filling the gaps between meals to prevent hunger or before that sweat session can make or break your dietary goals or your workout.

Choosing a snack with real food that's nutritious, provides energy and protein are an essential part of healthy eating. I love incorporating veggies and superfoods here as these are the foods give you unlimited energy and fiber that fills your up.

The protein shakes in this section are meal replacements and a simple way to boost you daily protein and nutrition. A rich and creamy smoothie can be a delicious way to start the day or as a meal replacement.

Don't fear protein powders ladies as whey protein is a perfect protein and isn't just for bodybuilders! It contains all the essential amino acids for a daily diet. It also boosts the immune system by increasing your body's production of glutathione, a powerful antioxidant essential for helping detoxification.

I use collagen protein a couple times per week and then chose a certified organic grass fed whey protein without any added ingredients for easier digestion and higher quality protein.

These are my go-to snacks and protein shakes to give you that fuel and satiation you need, in small amounts, to keep you going!

Garlic Chickpeas

Ingredients

2 x 15 oz cans......... chickpeas, organic
1/2 cup .... parsley, fresh, chopped
1 tbsp .... olive oil
2 tsp.................... garlic powder
1/4 tsp .... salt
1/2 tsp .... pepper

Spicy & Sweet Crispy Chickpeas

Ingredients

2 x 15 oz cans..... chickpeas, organic
2 tbsp .... olive oil
1 tsp .... garlic salt
1 tsp .... cumin

1 tsp .... chili powder
1/2 tsp .... cayenne
1 tsp .... stevia

Preparation

1. Preheat oven to 400F

2. Rinse, drain and dry chickpeas (make sure to thoroughly dry them so they come out crispy!).

4. Add chickpeas, oil and spices to a bowl and mix

5. Add to baking tray and bake for 40 mins (tossing every 20 min). If they aren't crispy and golden brown after 30 minutes, cook for 10 -15 minutes longer.

6. Once golden brown, remove from oven, and pile into a bowl for serving. Enjoy as a snack, on top of a salad, soup or bowl.

RYFIT TIP:
A great option for a portable snack. Store in an airtight container for the week!

Nutrition Facts
Servings: **3**
Calories Per Serving: **150**
Macros:
Protein: 13.5g
Total Carbs: 32g (6g Fiber)
Fat: 11g

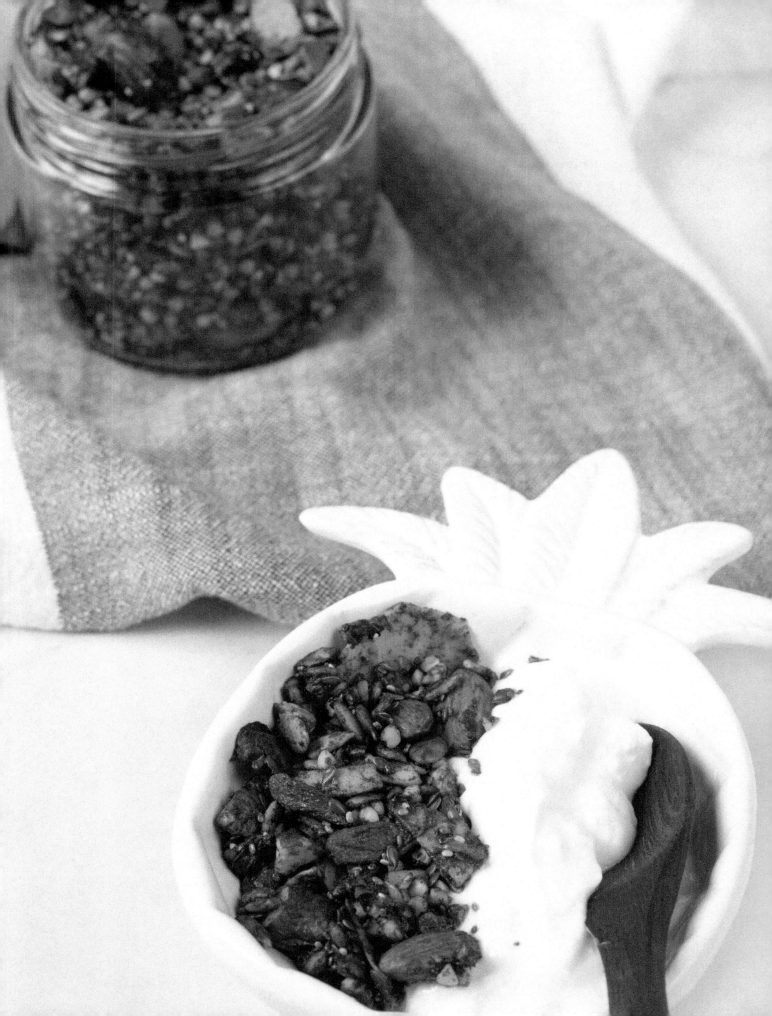

Ry's Homemade Hormone-Balancing Granola

I avoided granola my entire life because store-bought brands are loaded with sugar and full of poor quality ingredients - hence the inspiration for this recipe! Packed with hormone-balancing seeds, nuts, superfoods, fatty acids and adaptogens, this gluten and sugar free granola adds a satisfying crunch as a topper to your yogurt or pancakes.

Ingredients

1/2 cup ...... almonds, raw

1/2 cup ...... hazelnuts, raw

1/2 cup ...... sunflower seeds, raw

1/2 cup ...... flaxseeds, ground

1/4 cup ...... chia seeds

1/4 cup ...... goji berries

1/4 cup ..... pumpkin seeds

1 cup .... unsweetened coconut flakes

1 cup .... buckwheat groats

(may also use gluten free oats)

2 tbsp ...... cacao powder, raw

2 tbsp ...... coconut oil, melted

2 tbsp ...... sugar free maple syrup

1 tbsp .... maca

1 tsp .... salt

Preparation

1. Heat oven to 350 degrees Fahrenheit

2. Combine buckwheat, hazelnuts, almonds, dates, flax seeds, chia seeds, sunflower seeds, and coconut flakes in a bowl.

3. In a separate bowl, combine melted coconut, maple, cacao, maca, and salt. Pour the mixture over the seed/nut mix, and stir to combine.

4. Line a baking sheet with parchment paper, and spread the mixture evenly onto the sheet. Bake for 10 minutes.

5. Remove baking sheet from the oven, and break up the granola. Allow to cool completely before putting in an airtight container.

6. This will last in the refrigerator for two weeks (if you don't devour it before then!)

Nutrition Facts	Macros:
Servings: **10**	**Protein: 8g**
Calories Per Serving: **277**	**Total Carbs: 20.5g (8g Fiber)**
	Fat: 19g

Sweet Potato Hummus

This is a favorite of my entire family as it fuels our active, healthy lifestyle. It's brilliant orange and bursting with flavor, both savory and sweet. I eat it with nearly everything: bite-sized vegetables, as a substitute for mayonnaise or a dip with seed crackers.

Ingredients

1/2 cup ...... sweet potato
1 tbsp .... chipotle chili, chopped
2 tbsp .... lemon juice
1 tbsp .... olive oil

Preparation

Combine all ingredients in a blender or food processor and process until smooth.

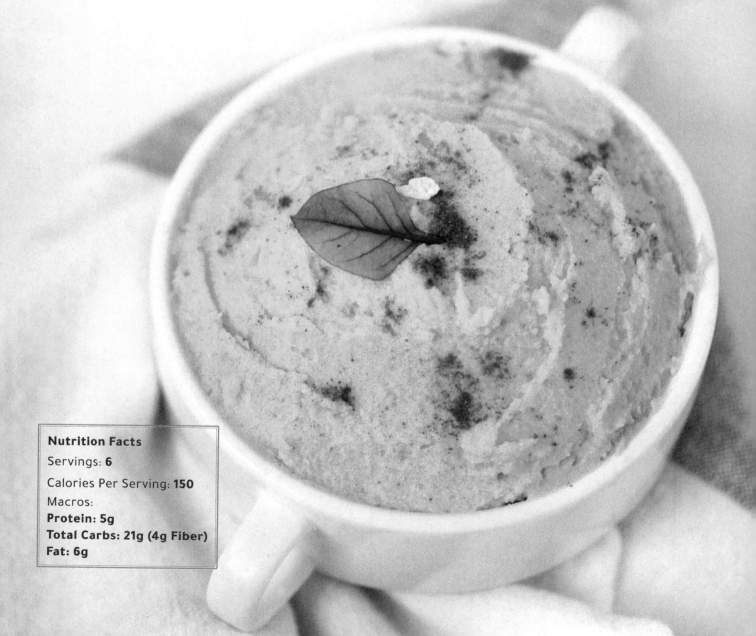

Nutrition Facts
Servings: **6**
Calories Per Serving: **150**
Macros:
Protein: 5g
Total Carbs: 21g (4g Fiber)
Fat: 6g

Collagen Beet Hummus

HOT pink. Lemony with a kick of garlic. Super creamy and flavorful. Full of vitamins and minerals. Beets help to activate your liver enzymes and, boost your livers detoxifying function. Collagen powder provides a punch of protein plus helps support skin, muscles, bone and connective tissue. The perfect dip for a gluten free cracker, veggies or a spread. What's not to love?!

Ingredients

1	beet, small, roasted, peeled
2 x 15 oz cans	chickpeas, organic
1	lemon, large, zested
¼ cup	collagen powder
½	lemon, large, juiced
¼ tsp	salt & pepper
2	garlic, cloves, large, minced
2 tbsp	tahini
1/4 cup	olive oil

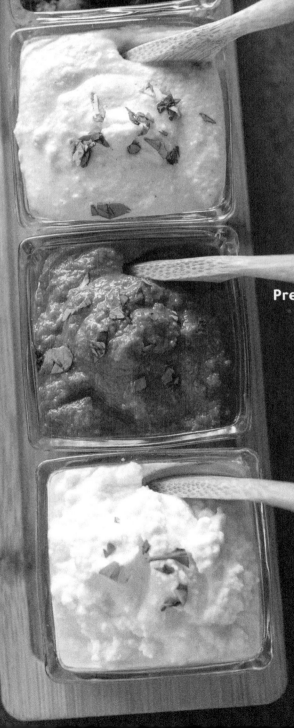

Preparation

1. Once your beet is cooled and peeled, quarter it and place it in your food processor. Blend until only small bits remain.

2. Add remaining ingredients except for olive oil and blend until smooth.

3. Drizzle in olive oil as the hummus is mixing.

4. Taste and adjust seasonings as needed, adding more salt, lemon juice, or olive oil if needed. If it's too thick, add a bit of water.

5. Will keep in the fridge for up to a week.

Nutrition Facts	Macros:
Servings: **6**	Protein: **9g**
	Total Carbs: **19g** (5g Fiber)
Calories Per Serving: **225**	Fat: **14g**

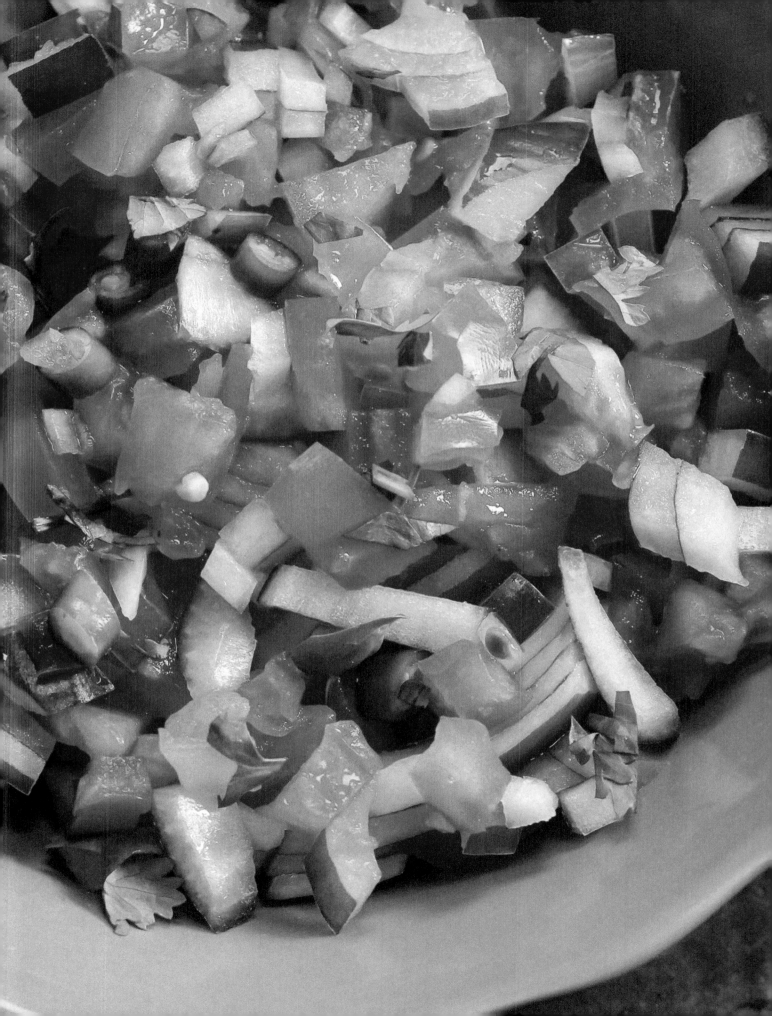

Metabolic Boosting Salsa

It doesn't get any more authentic than this! Credit goes to my amazing partner, Marcelo, as this is his family recipe. Simple to make and loaded with the fresh flavors of Mexico, this is a staple in our house for topping eggs, tortillas, healthy totopos (tortilla chips!), and a perfect compliment to guacamole. Loaded with flavor not calories... once you make this fresh you'll never go back to store-bought salsa!

Ingredients

1/3 cup	cilantro, fresh		1/8 tsp	salt & pepper
4 cloves	garlic, large		1/8 tsp	cumin
5	tomatoes, medium		1/8 tsp	cayenne pepper
1	onion, medium			
1-2	jalapeno peppers			

*optional for spice

Preparation

1. Boil the tomatoes with garlic & onion until soft.

2. If you're using jalapeño peppers: In a preheated frying pan, add 1 tsp of olive oil and fry the jalapeño peppers until soft.

3. Add all of this to a blender or food processor with salt, pepper, cumin, cayenne pepper, and fresh cilantro.

4. Taste the finished product to determine if you have enough jalapeño for your desired heat level. Remember you can always add more but you can't take it out once you've added it!

5. Serve cold and store it in the fridge in an airtight jar - it stays fresh for up to a week!

Nutrition Facts
Servings: **10**
Calories Per Serving: **15**
Macros:
Protein: 0g
Total Carbs: .5g
Fat: 0g

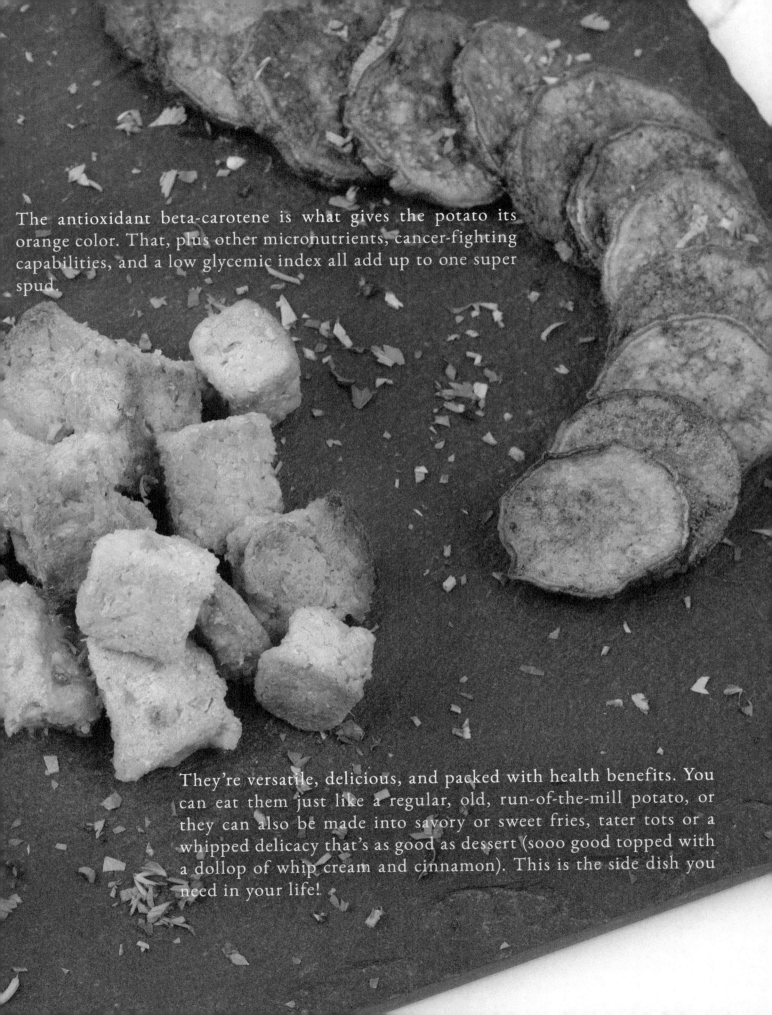

The antioxidant beta-carotene is what gives the potato its orange color. That, plus other micronutrients, cancer-fighting capabilities, and a low glycemic index all add up to one super spud.

They're versatile, delicious, and packed with health benefits. You can eat them just like a regular, old, run-of-the-mill potato, or they can also be made into savory or sweet fries, tater tots or a whipped delicacy that's as good as dessert (sooo good topped with a dollop of whip cream and cinnamon). This is the side dish you need in your life!

Sweet Baked Fries

Ingredients

2 .... sweet potatoes, medium

1 tbsp .... peanut oil

1 tbsp....... olive oil

1 tsp .... cinnamon

1/4 tsp ...... cayenne pepper

1/4 tsp ...... salt

1 tbsp .... monk fruit sweetener

Savory Baked Fries

Ingredients

2.............. sweet potatoes, medium

2 tbsp .... olive oil

1 tsp .... paprika, dried

1 tsp .... oregano, dried

1 tsp .... cumin, ground

1/4 tsp ...... salt

1/4 tsp ...... pepper

Preparation (both recipes)

1. Preheat the oven to 400 degrees Fahrenheit. Clean and peel the sweet potatoes, cut into ½ inch strips, pat them dry and place in a bowl

2. Combine the oils with herbs and spices. Pour over the sweet potatoes and toss to coat thoroughly. Sprinkle with toppings.

3. Spread wedges in a single layer on a large baking sheet and bake for 10 minutes. Flip and increase the temperature to 425, flip every 10 minutes (30 minutes in total) or until they are tender and start to darken in color.

Nutrition Facts

Servings: **4**

Calories Per Serving: **145**

Macros:

Protein: 1g

Total Carbs: 15g (2g Fiber)

Fat: 9g

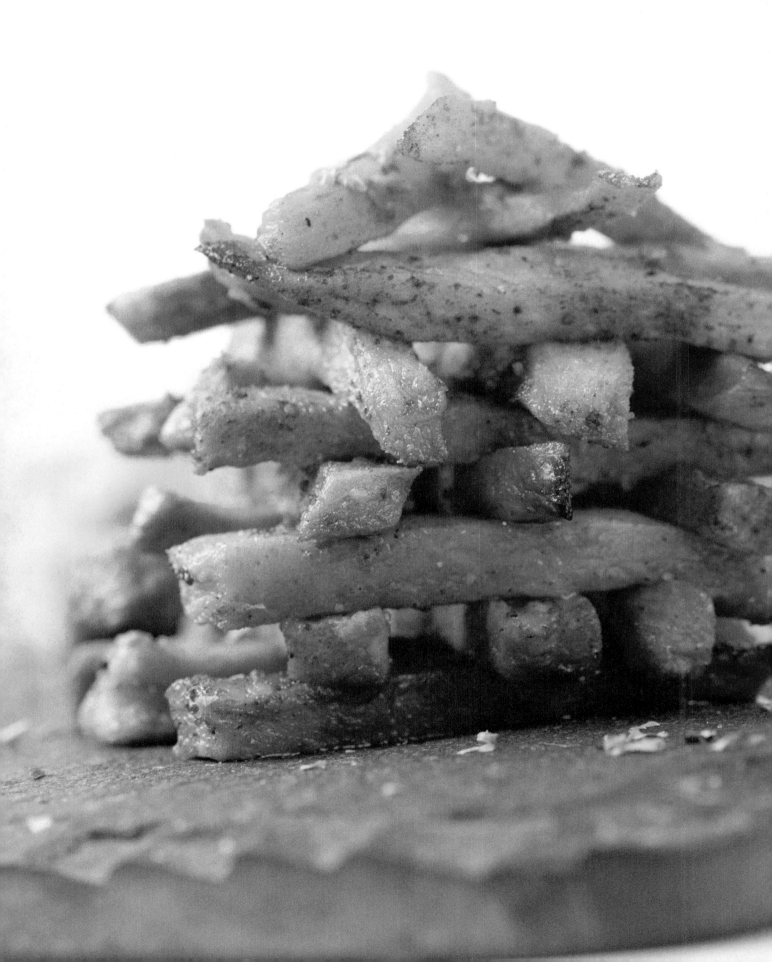

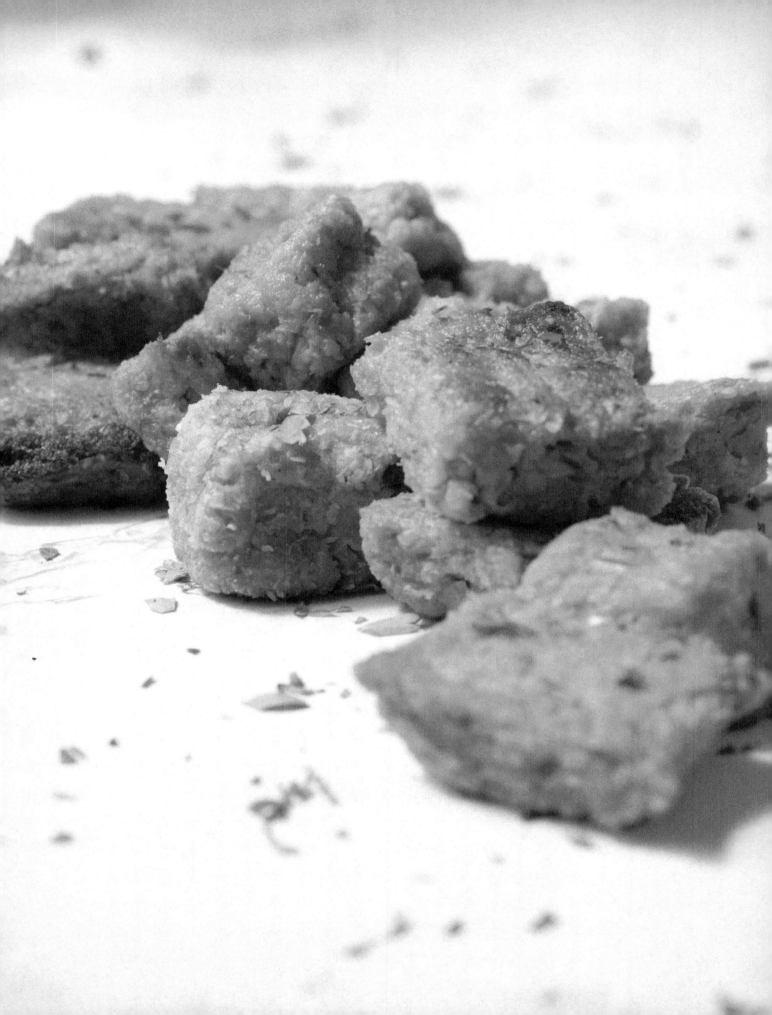

Sweet Potato Tater Tots

Ingredients

1 cup .... sweet potatoes, mashed

1/8 cup...... egg white

1/8 tsp ...... pepper

1/4 tsp ...... salt

1/2 tsp ...... garlic powder

1/3 cup...... onions, chopped

1/3 cup...... oat flour

Preparation

1. Preheat oven to 375 degrees Fahrenheit. In a bowl, mix all ingredients together until well combined

2. Form about 1.5-2 tsp of potato mixture into "tater tot" shapes and transfer to a baking sheet lined with foil and sprayed. Spray tops of tots with olive oil cooking spray. Bake for 20-25 minutes, until browned and crisp on top. Feel free to broil for the last minute to brown up if desired.

Nutrition Facts
Servings: **2 (15 tater tots)**
Calories Per Serving: **150**
Macro
Protein: 6g
Total Carbs: 19g (3g Fiber)
Fat: 1g

Sweet Potato Soufflé

Ingredients

3.............. sweet potatoes, large

3/4 cup ..... unsweetened dairy free milk

1 tbsp .... honey

2 tbsp .... ghee

3.............. egg whites

1/4 tsp ...... cinnamon

2 tsp......... stevia

1/8 tsp ...... nutmeg

1/8 tsp ...... cilli powder

1/8 tsp ...... red pepper flakes, crushed

1/4 cup...... pecans or walnuts, chopped

1/8 cup...... sugar free maple syrup

Preparation

1. Preheat oven to 350 degrees Fahrenheit.

2. Boil sweet potatoes and remove skin. Put potatoes into a blender or food processor.

3. In a bowl beat egg whites until soft peaks form and place aside.

4. Add ghee, honey, cinnamon, nutmeg, cilli powder, red pepper flakes, almond milk, syrup and egg whites to the sweet potato in the blender or food processor and blend into a creamy mixture.

5. Transfer mixture to a casserole dish or ramekins, sprinkle with nuts and bake for 20-25 minutes (until egg is set).

Nutrition Facts

Servings: **5**

Calories Per Serving: **152**

Macros:

Protein: 6g

Total Carbs: 27g (4g Fiber)

Fat: 5g

RyFit Tip:

This is my all-time favorite way to prepare sweet potatoes. Top it with some sugar free syrup and it can double as a dessert!

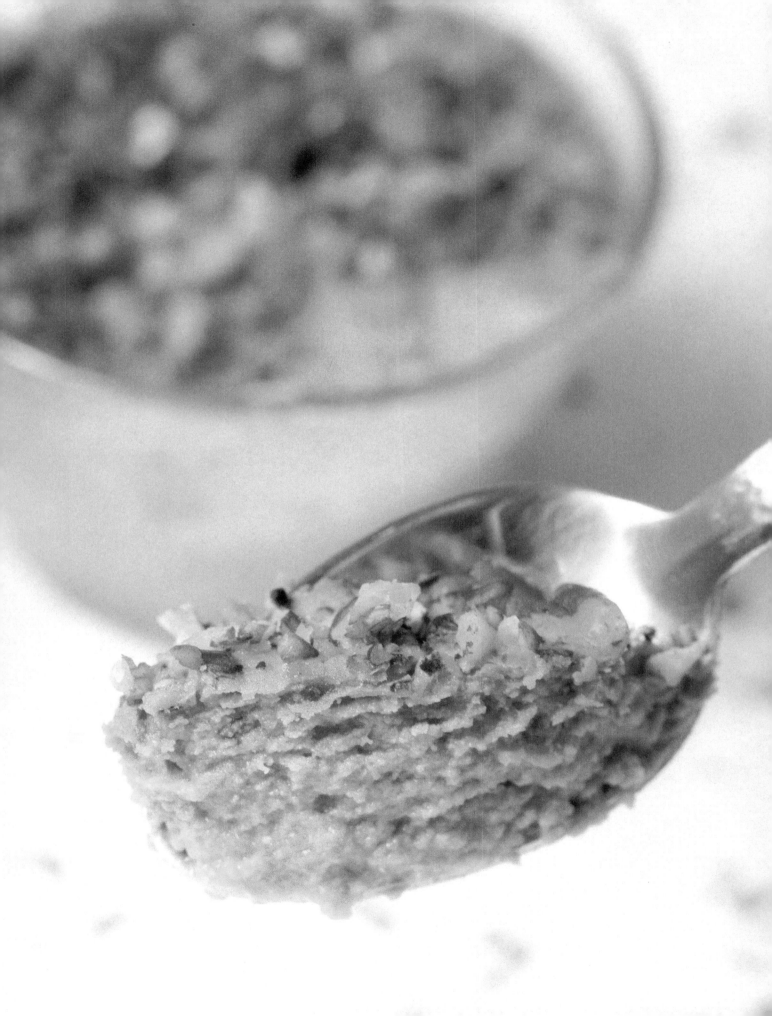

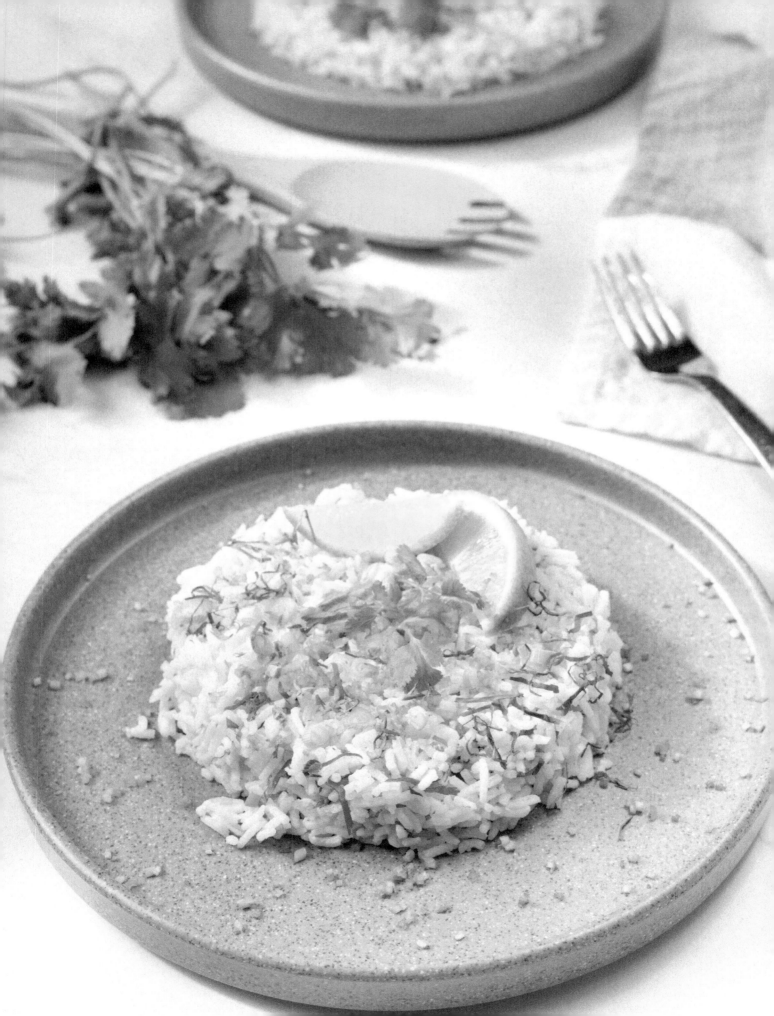

Coconut Basmati Rice

White basmati Rice has a low glycemic load (great for diabetics and healthy living) and I absolutely love the texture - this was my go-to carb as a fitness competitor. Fragrant and tropically flavored, this coconut rice makes a perfect side dish.

Ingredients

14 ounce ... **can light, organic, unsweetened coconut milk, well shaken**
*if you can't find then use unsweetened coconut milk in box
1 3/4 cups .. **water**

2 cups .... **basmati rice, white**
1 tsp .... **salt**
1 tsp .... **lime zest**
1/4 cup ...... **green onion, thinly sliced**
1/4 cup ...... **cilantro leaves, fresh, chopped**

Preparation

1. Measure out 1 ½ cups of the canned coconut milk and add to a medium saucepan (save the remaining coconut milk for later).

2. Add the water, rice and salt to the saucepan. Mix to combine. Bring the mixture to a boil, then cover, turn down the heat and simmer for about 15 to 20 minutes, until the liquid is absorbed and the rice is tender.

3. Turn off the heat, then let stand covered for 5 to 10 minutes untouched.

4. Fluff with a fork, stir in the lime zest, green onion, cilantro and remaining coconut milk. Let the rice stand uncovered for another 5 minutes, then serve!

Nutrition Facts
Servings: **4**
Calories Per Serving: **229**
Macros:
Protein: 1.5g
Total Carbs: 23g
Fat: 7g

Powerful Pomegranate Mint Quinoa

Pine nuts and pomegranate are a powerful combo. Pine nuts are energizers as they're packed with protein, iron, and magnesium and the antioxidant power of both of these will help keep your skin healthy and youthful - here's to aging well!

Ingredients

1 cup	quinoa, cooked
1/2 cup	pomegranate seeds
1 tbsp	mint, chopped
1 tbsp	parsley, chopped
2 tbsp	pine nuts, toasted
1/2	lemon juiced + zested
1/8 tsp	salt & pepper

Preparation

Add all ingredients to cooked quinoa and hand blend. Simple, so fresh and pretty - enjoy!

Nutrition Facts
Servings: **2**
Calories Per Serving: **190**
Macros:
Protein: 5g
Total Carbs: 21g (4g Fiber)
Fat: 8g

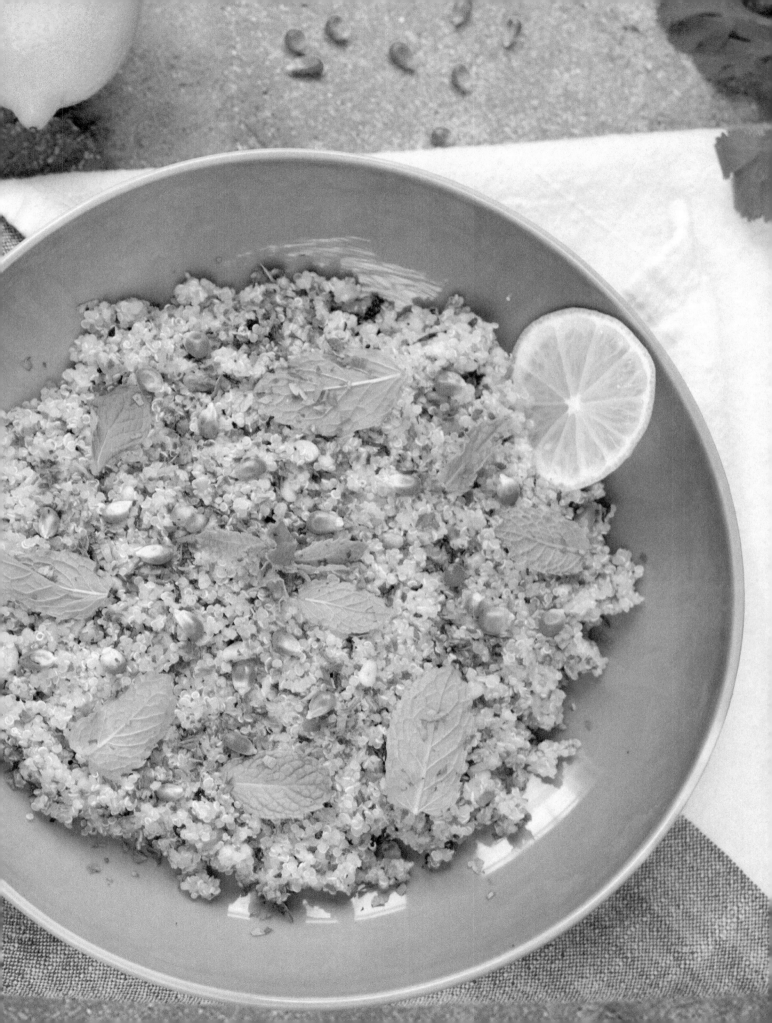

Three Bean & Mushroom Stew

Warning - this is not your average stew!
A vegan meal packed with flavor and nutrients plus it offers anti-inflammatory and immune boosting properties - make a double batch so you can keep some in the freezer.

Ingredients

3 tbsp ...... olive oil, avocado oil or ghee

2 lb .... mixed mushrooms
(cremini, oyster, chanterelles, shiitake the more variety, the more flavor),

3 .... shallots, diced

2 tbsp ...... tomato paste, low sodium, organic

2 tsp .... thyme leaves, fresh

2 tsp .... cumin, minced

2 tsp .... coriander

1 1/2 tsp .... cinnamon

1/8 tsp ...... allspice, ground

1 tsp .... salt

1 tsp .... pepper

1/2 cup ..... kidney beans

1/2 cup ..... black beans

1/2 cup ..... butter beans

6 cups ...... vegetable broth,
low sodium, or water with a squeeze of lime

Preparation

1. Heat oil in a large pot over medium-high heat. Add mushrooms and shallots and cook until slightly browned, about 10 minutes.

2. Sprinkle in tomato paste, thyme, cumin, coriander, cinnamon, and allspice. Sauté for 1 minute.

3. Stir in broth or water, salt, pepper, and beans. Bring mixture to a simmer over medium heat. Cook for 20 minutes or until slightly thickened. You can also add this to a crock pot and leave simmer on low for added flavor.

4. Remove soup from heat, and add a squeeze of lime, and enjoy.

Nutrition Facts
Servings: **6**
Calories Per Serving: **181**
Macros:
Protein: 10g
Total Carbs: 16g (4g Fiber)
Fat: 9g

Quinoa Chilli

Traditional Chili gets an upgrade when 'superfood' quinoa is stacked with beans. A perfect, plant-based meal a couple of hours before sweating to fuel a long workout or a healthy, hearty lunch option. Quinoa and beans pack a serious punch of fiber, protein, iron and magnesium - a nutritious and delicious choice!

Ingredients

1/2 cup .... quinoa, uncooked

1 cup .... water

1 15-oz can ...... black beans, organic

1 tsp .... chili powder

1 tsp .... curry powder

1 tsp .... cinnamon

2 .... green onions, diced

1/2 cup .... tomatoes, diced

1/4 tsp .... stevia (to taste)

Preparation

1. Bring quinoa and water to a boil and simmer for 15 minute (until germ separates).

2. In a separate pot simmer black bean together with seasonings for 10 minutes. Allow beans to cool and thicken for 5 minutes.

3. Combine quinoa and bean mixture together. Top with tomatoes and green onions and serve.

Nutrition Facts
Servings: **6**
Calories Per Serving: **395**
Macros:
Protein: 22g
Total Carbs: 70g (19g Fiber)
Fat: 2g

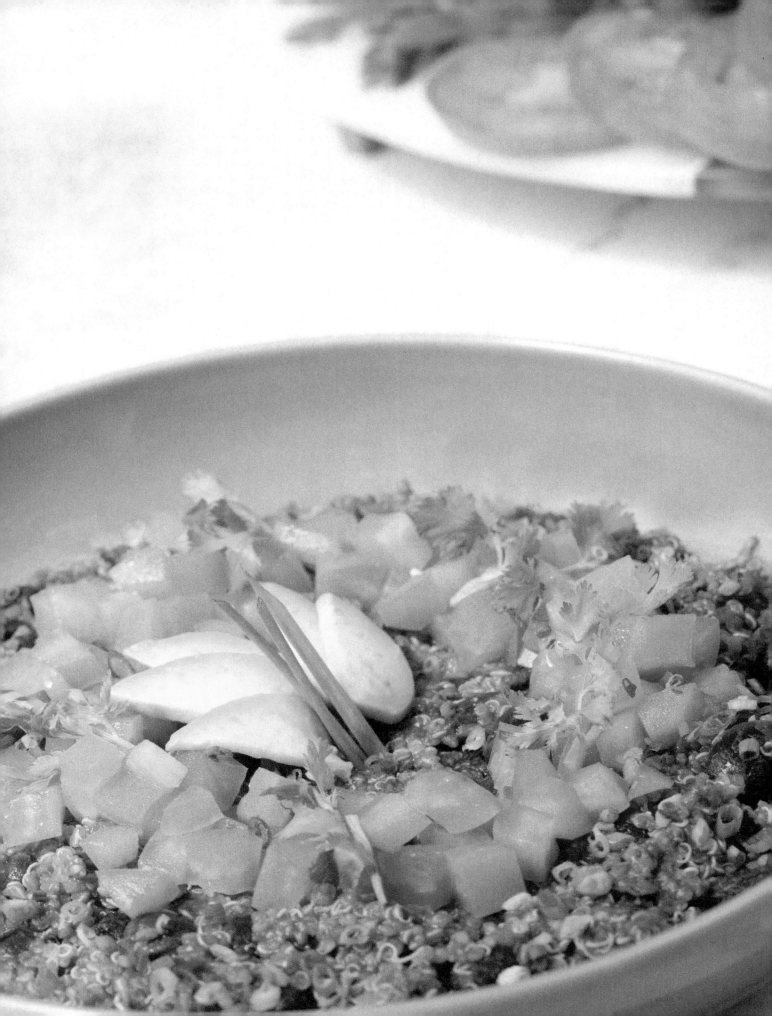

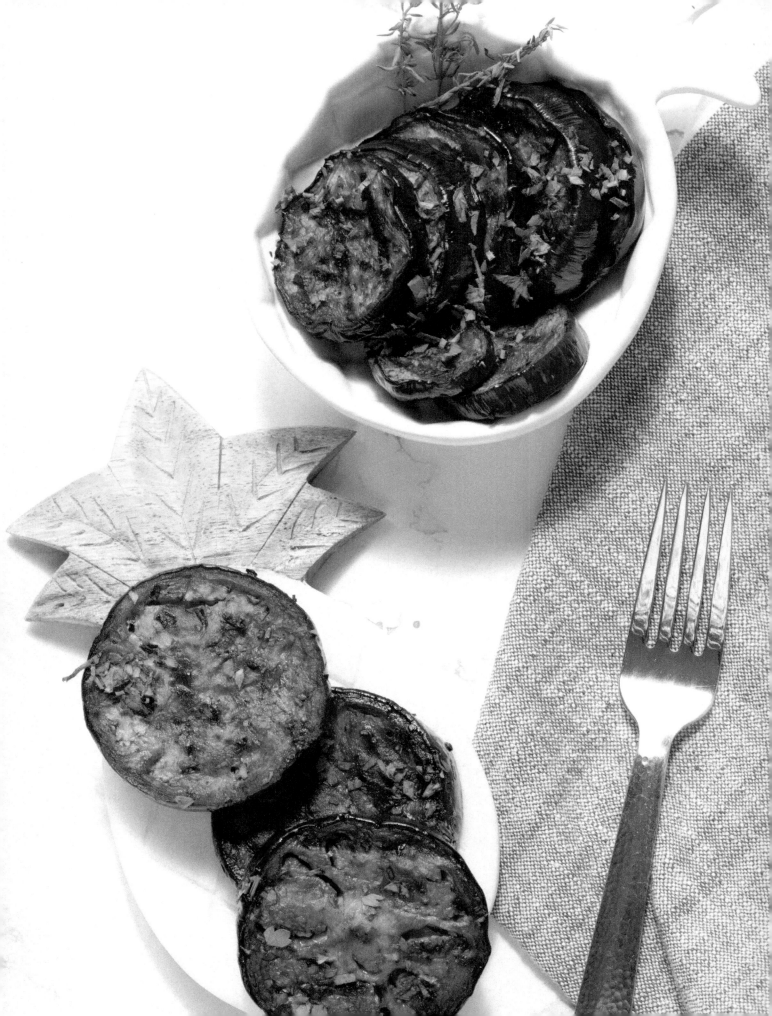

Marinated Grilled Eggplant

Eggplant is an excellent source of potassium, which aids in maintaining muscle strength, contraction and water balance. And on the grill is always a hit!

Ingredients

2 tbsp .... balsamic vinegar

1 tbsp .... olive oil

1 .... garlic clove, minced

1 .... eggplant, medium-sized

Preparation

1. Mix balsamic vinegar, olive oil and garlic

2. Cut eggplant into ½-inch thick slices

3. Place eggplant slices into the marinade and coat. Allow to sit for 1 hour

4. Preheat grill and place eggplant on the grill until lightly browned, about 4 minutes.
Flip and brown the other side.

Nutrition Facts
Servings: **4**
Calories Per Serving: **70**
Macros:
Protein: 1g
Total Carbs: 10g (4g Fiber)
Fat: 3g

Healthy Cheesy Potato Soup

Don't let the list of ingredients scare you - the steps are simple and you only need one pot. Comfort food made healthy, this soup can be made on the stove, in the slow cooker, Crockpot or instant pot. All the flavor of regular loaded baked potato soup with WAY better ingredients - and 1/4 the calories and fat you'd normally find in it! This soup is a winner.

Ingredients

3 cups.......	broth, beef, chicken or vegetable, organic, low sodium
1/3 cup......	gluten free flour
2 cups.......	unsweetened dairy free milk
2 lbs	Yukon gold potatoes, diced
1 tsp	salt
1/2 tsp	thyme, dried
1/4 tsp	pepper
1/8 tsp	red pepper flakes, crushed
1/2 cup......	cheddar cheese, sharp, shredded, organic
1/2 cup......	Greek yogurt, low fat or fat free
Toppings: ..	chopped bacon, shredded organic cheese, green onions, greek yogurt

Preparation

1. In a large pot, cook the bacon over medium high heat, until crispy. Transfer the bacon to a plate with a paper towel to soak up some of the grease.

2. Add ghee to the pot and melt over medium heat. Cook the onion, carrot, and celery until tender. Add in the garlic and cook until fragrant.

3. Stir in the flour and cook for 1 to 2 minutes, stirring occasionally. This will help thicken up the soup. Add the broth, milk, potatoes, salt, thyme, pepper, and crushed red pepper flakes. Stir until combined.

4. Bring to a boil and then reduce the heat to low. Cover and cook for 10 to 15 minutes or until potatoes are soft. Make sure you stir the soup often so the potatoes don't stick to the bottom of the pot.

5. Stir in the cheese and greek yogurt. SO creamy!! Taste and season with salt & pepper, to taste. If you're lactose intolerant you can simply leave the cheese out. Drizzle with cheese, yogurt, bacon and chives.

Nutrition Facts
Servings: **4**
Calories Per Serving: **245**
Macros:
Protein: 14.5g
Total Carbs: 25g (7g Fiber)
Fat: 7g

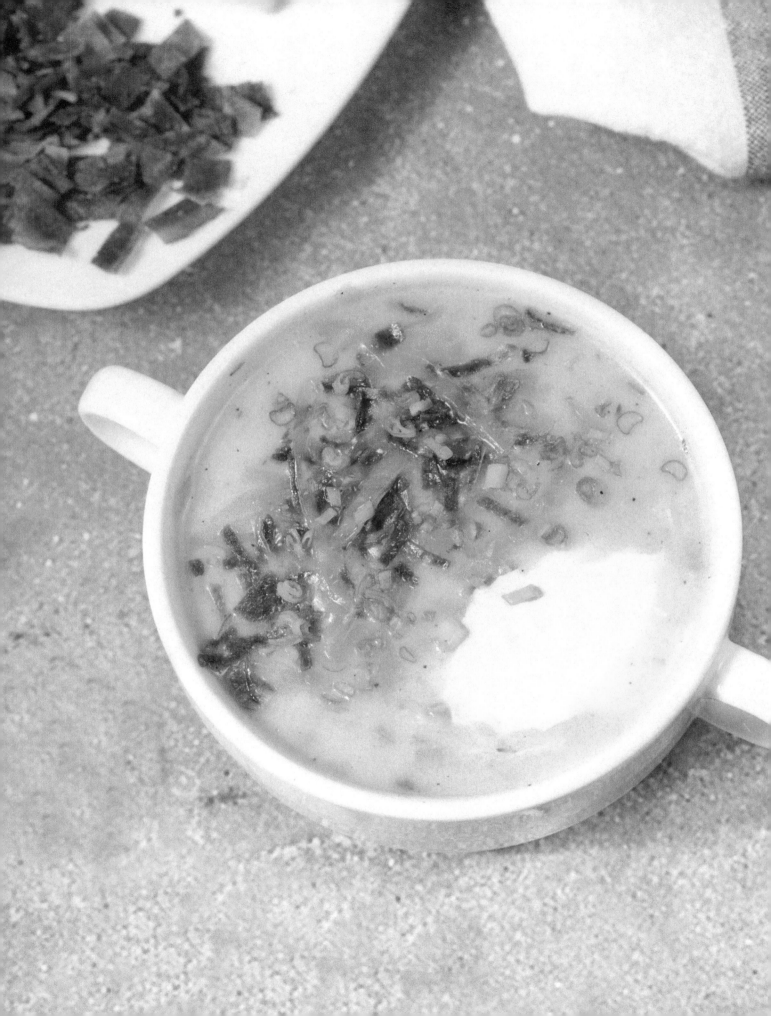

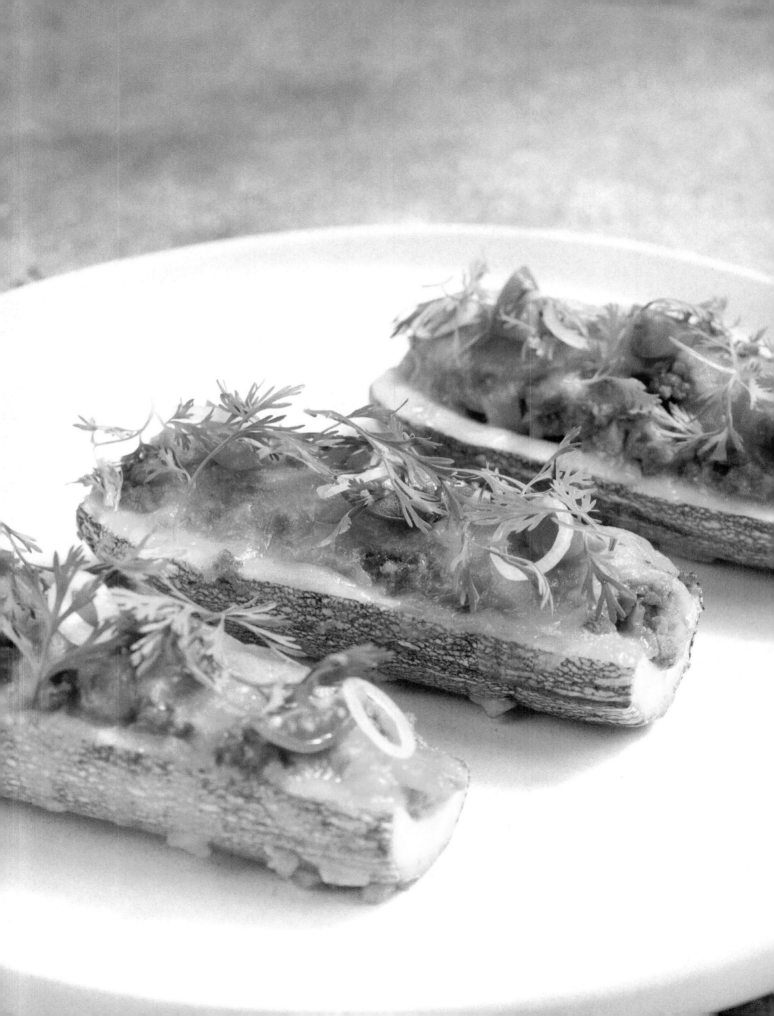

Zucchini Tacos

Don't let the steps fool you - these are easy to make and a fun way to put healthy twist on taco night. This recipe is low-carb, paleo, keto and so satisfying!

Ingredients

4 .... zucchini, whole, medium	1 cup .... cauliflower rice, (i buy mine pre-riced)
1 cup .... salsa (page 175)	2 .... garlic cloves, chopped
1 tbsp .... olive oil	1 bell .... pepper, chopped
1/2 cup ..... onion, chopped	1/2 tsp ...... salt & pepper
12 oz .... ground beef, extra lean	1/2 cup ..... cheddar cheese, shredded, organic
2 tbsp ...... taco seasoning, no added preservatives	1/4 cup ..... cilantro, chopped *optional
	1/4 cup ..... diced cherry tomatoes *optional

Preparation

```
Nutrition Facts
Servings: 8
Calories Per Serving: 245
Macros:
Protein: 26g
Total Carbs: 4.5g (1g Fiber)
Fat: 12g
```

1. Pre-heat oven to 350F.

2. Trim the top and bottom of zucchini off. Lay the zucchini flat and slice in half lengthwise. Repeat with all four zucchini.

3. Using a spoon, scoop the center of the zucchini out leaving 1/4 inch wall around the bottom and sides of the zucchini. Repeat with each zucchini half.

4. Reserve 1 cup of the zucchini meat from the center of the zucchini and give it a rough chop. We will use this in the filling.

5. Add a thin layer of salsa to the bottom of a baking and lay the zucchini boats on top. You may need two dishes to fit all of the zucchini.

6. In a large non stick skillet, heat olive oil. Once the oil is hot, add in the onion along with a pinch of salt. When it's translucent add in ground beef. Season with salt and break up into crumbles. Add taco seasoning and stir to coat.

7. Next, add in cauliflower rice, garlic, bell pepper and zucchini meat. Season with a little more salt & pepper and stir. Pour in remaining salsa, stir everything together, and simmer for 5-10 minutes. Turn off the heat and allow it to cool until it's easy to handle.

8. Divide the mixture evenly amongst all 8 zucchini boat halves and then sprinkle each half with shredded cheddar cheese.

9. Bake for 25 minutes or until the cheese has melted and the zucchini is tender. Top with fresh tomatoes and cilantro and enjoy!

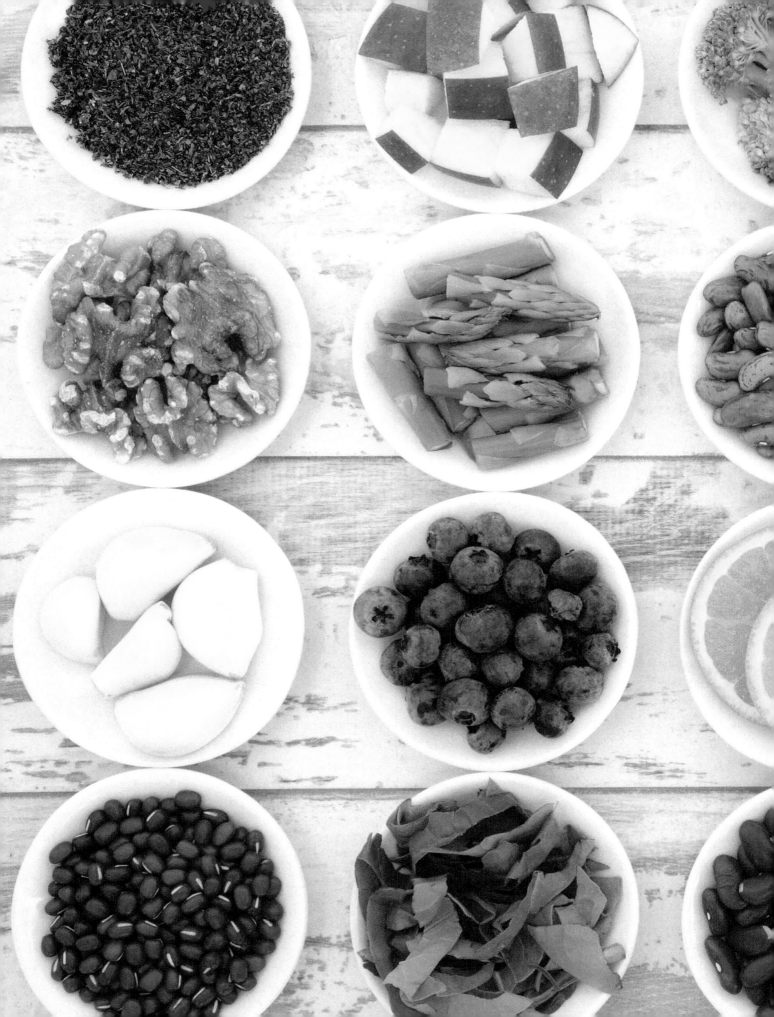

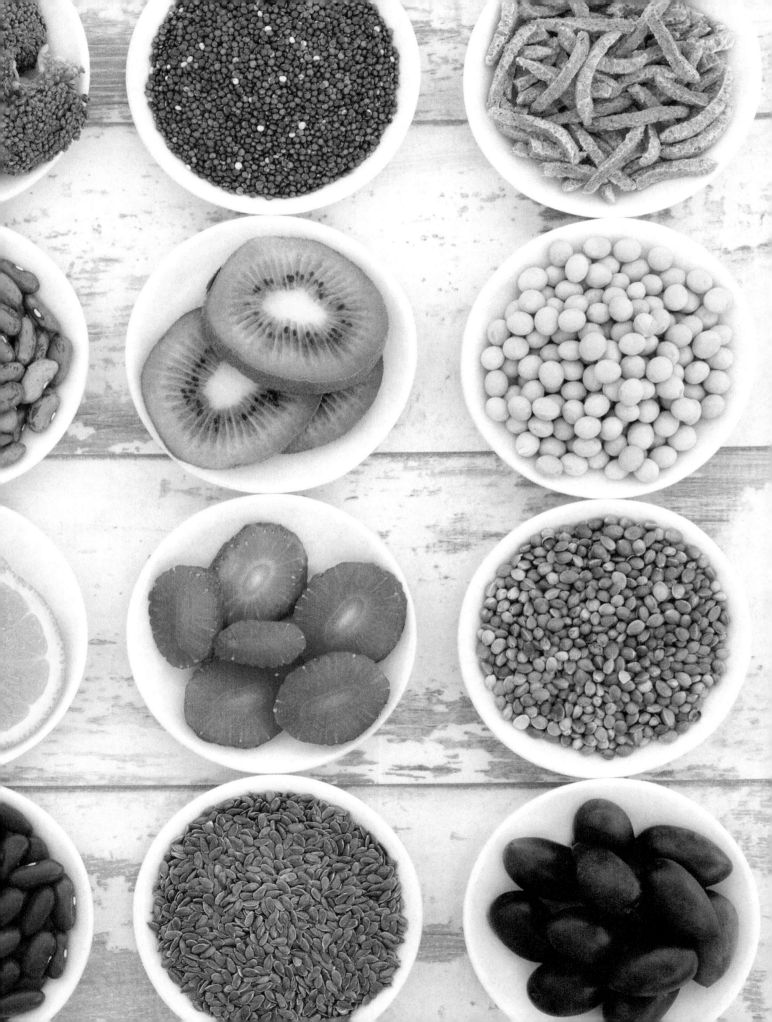

Quinoa & Bean Salad

This Quinoa Black Bean Salad is bursting with colorful ingredients. It's a big bowl of clean, plant-based, hearty ingredients tossed in a zesty garlic lime vinaigrette. A quick and easy recipe that comes together in 20 minutes! Put that leftover quinoa to good use and enjoy it for days as a light lunch or a side dish for a crowd.

Ingredients

2 x 5oz ...... white tuna, cans, in water, drained

1 x 15oz ..... black beans, can, drained and rinsed

1/2 cup ...... carrot juice, fresh
(or buy with no added sugar)

3 tbsp .... olive oil

1 .... lemon, freshly juice

1/4 tsp ...... pepper

Preparation

1. Heat a large saucepan over medium heat. Add quinoa and drizzle of olive oil, toast it, shaking pan often, until fragrant and beginning to pop (3-4 minutes). Add 2 cups of water and cover, simmering over medium-low heat until tender, about 12 minutes. Set aside to cool and then fluff with a fork.

2. Steam or boil asparagus until tender.

3. In a large bowl, toss together quinoa, asparagus, tuna, black beans, yellow pepper, cherry tomatoes, parsley, scallions, walnuts and dried fruit. In a separate bowl, whisk together carrot juice, olive oil, lemon juice, garlic, cumin, salt & pepper. Pour carrot juice mixture over quinoa mixture, toss and voila!

Nutrition Facts

Servings: **6**

Calories Per Serving: **387**

Macros:
Protein: 22g
Total Carbs: 44g (9g Fiber)
Fat: 16g

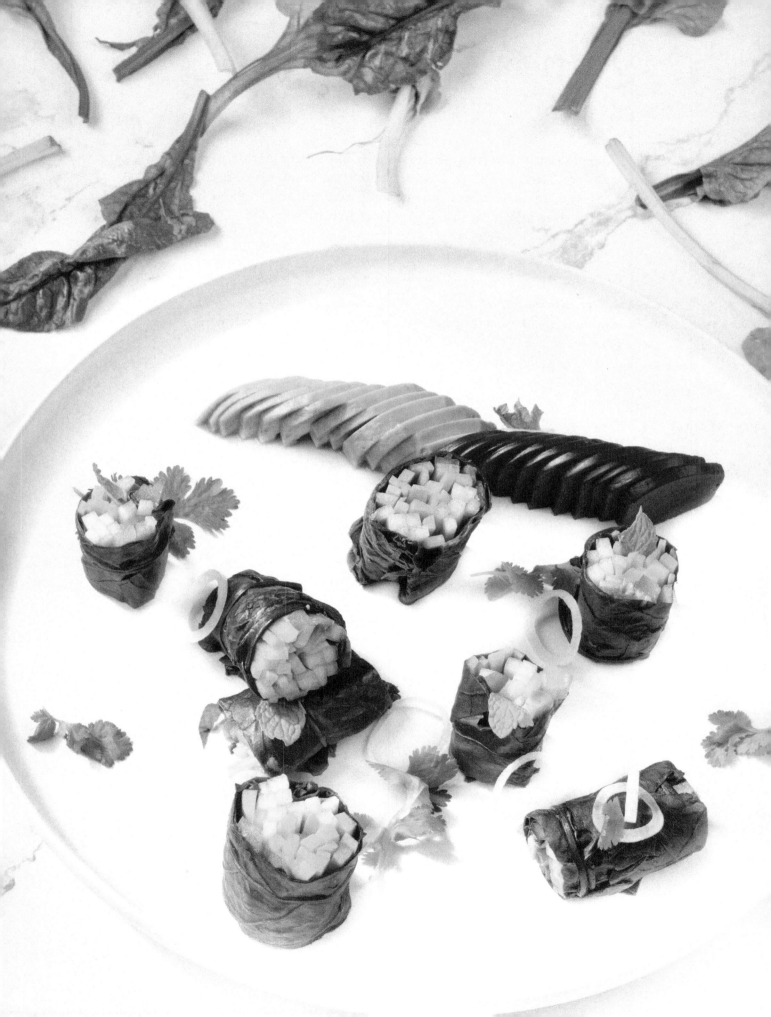

Collard Green Rainbow Wrap

There are so many reasons to love these collard green wraps. They're loaded with fiber and liver-loving veggies, and they're also gluten-free, dairy-free, plant-based, delicious, and most importantly, FUN! The wraps aren't hard to fold, and once you have your fillings on hand they take minutes to make. Perfect for a light lunch or dinner.

Ingredients

4 .... collard green leaves

2 .... beets, steamed

1 .... red bell pepper, sliced

1 .... yellow bell pepper, sliced

1/2 cup ...... fermented vegetables
            (carrots or kimchi)

1 .... carrot, sliced into 4 inch strips

2 .... radish, sliced into strips

1 .... cucumber,
            sliced into 4 inch strips

2 .... green onions, whites and greens
            thinly sliced

1 .... avocado, thinly sliced

1 .... bunch of cilantro, chopped

1 .... bunch mint, leaves

Preparation

1. Bring a large pot of water to a boil. Make an ice bath in a large bowl.

2. Using tongs, dip each collard green into the boiling water for a few seconds, until bright green. Transfer to ice bath, and repeat with each collard green leaf. Remove leaves from water, and pat dry. Cut the base of the stem off, and shave as much of the remaining stem off to make them more pliable.

3. Pile the vegetables on top of the collard green, perpendicular to the base of the stem.

4. Roll one end of the collard greens over the fillings, lengthwise, then fold in the ends, and continue to roll. Place seam side down, slice in half, and put on a serving plate.

5. Dip collard green wraps into the Ah-mazing Almond Butter Sauce on page 316 and enjoy!

Nutrition Facts

Servings: **2**

Calories Per Serving: **250**

Macros:

Protein: 6.5g

Total Carbs: 31g (12.5g Fiber)

Fat: 14.5g

Chickpea Power Patties

These patties make an amazing vegan chickpea burger patty, they work perfectly as a filling in a wrap or as a salad topping and make a great portable snack - just adjust the size of the patty for what you need.

Ingredients

4 .... green onions, chopped

1/2 cup ...... mushrooms, diced

2 x 15-oz .... garbanzo beans, organic, canned, undrained, low sodium

6 .... garlic cloves, fresh, chopped

1/4 cup ...... onion, chopped

3 tbsp .... cilantro, fresh, chopped

3 tsp .... parsley, fresh, chopped

3 tbsp .... curry powder

1 tsp .... cumin, ground

1 cup .... gluten free oats

3 .... egg whites

Preparation

1. Preheat oven to 375 F.

2. Heat a non-stick pan or lightly sprayed pan on medium. Add green onions and mushrooms and cook until tender.

3. Blend the undrained beans, garlic and onions in a food processor until creamy.

4. In a bowl, mix the bean mixture with the green onions and mushrooms. Add herbs, spices, bread crumbs, egg whites and mix well.

5. Spray a baking sheet with cooking spray. Form the mixture into balls and flatten. Place in the oven for 20 minutes or until brown.

Nutrition Facts
Servings: **16**
Calories Per Serving: **90**
Macros:
Protein: 5g
Total Carbs: 14g (3g Fiber)
Fat: 1g

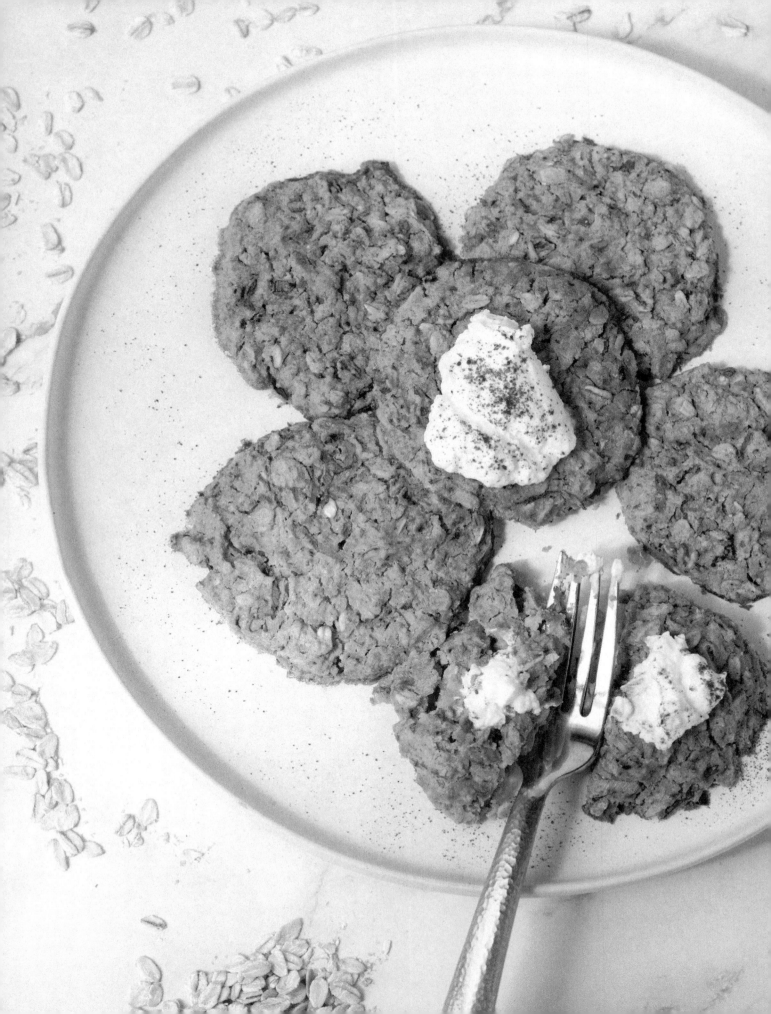

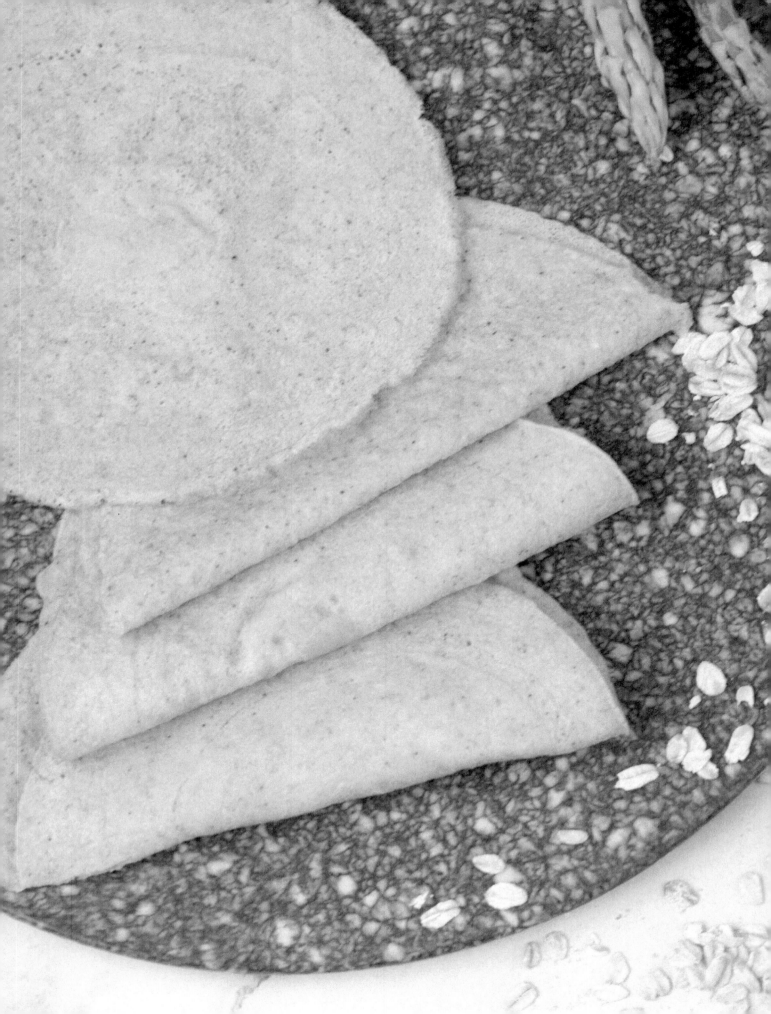

Gluten Free Protein Tortillas

Meet the tortilla from Mexican healthy heaven! I love this recipe because the tortilla is actually packed with protein itself - plus loads of fiber, which make these extremely filling. These are my go-to tortillas for tacos, wraps or mini crepes. Your kids will love them with nut butter and banana as a snack!

Ingredients

1/8 cup...... oat flour

1 tbsp .... coconut flour

1.............. whole egg

3.............. egg whites

1/4 cup...... unsweetened dairy free milk

1/4 tsp ...... salt & pepper

1 tsp .... garlic powder

Preparation

1. Hand mix all ingredients in a large bowl and pour into a large, sprayed frying pan on low-medium heat.

You want a small frying pan and pour your batter thin to create a tortilla for a taco.

Once it starts to bubble flip it and cook until golden brown.

Nutrition Facts

Servings: **2 tortilla**

Calories Per Serving: **110**

Macros:

Protein: 10g

Total Carbs: 8.5g (3.5g Fiber)

Fat: 3.5g

RyFit Tip:

Make a big batch and freeze them to save time. Once cooled place them between parchment paper and store in an air-tight container.

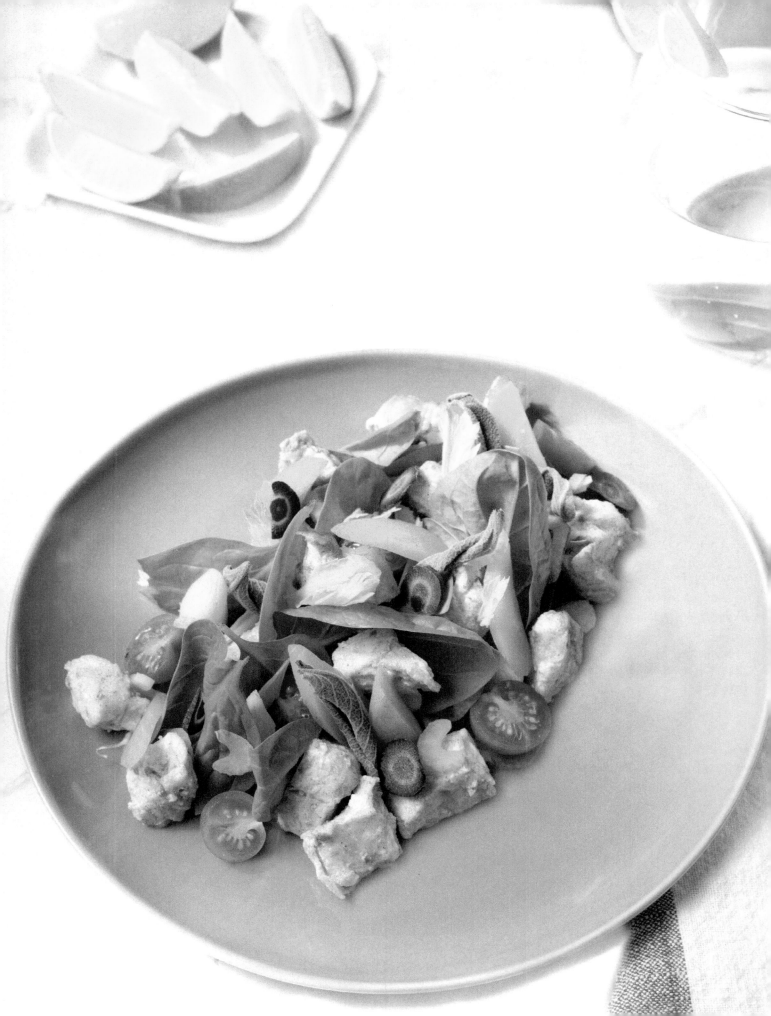

SEAFOOD

Heart-healthy, nutrient-dense proteins that make every meal delicious and balanced. Seafood boasts thyroid-supporting nutrients iodine and selenium, and is also our best source of omega-3 fatty acids. Always opt for wild-caught, low-mercury sustainable raised seafood.

Lemon Garlic Sweet Salmon

This flavorful lemon garlic salmon recipe makes a delicious, protein-packed dinner served with your favorite salad or side dishes, and the marinade is perfect for any protein. I always use sugar free maple syrup instead of honey to eliminate the sugar without reducing the sweetness or flavor factor!

Ingredients

1 lb .... wild salmon, skin on

2 tbsp .... ghee, melted

2 tbsp .... sugar free maple syrup

1 tsp .... dijon mustard, preferably grainy dijon

1/2 tbsp ..... lemon, fresh juiced

1 .... lemon zest

1/2 tsp ...... garlic powder
(or 3 cloves garlic, minced)

1/4 tsp ...... salt & pepper

Preparation

1. Preheat your oven to 400 degrees F.

2. For the marinade, combine whisk all of the ingredients in a bowl and generously season the salmon.

3. Line a large baking sheet with parchment paper or lightly coat with olive, coconut or avocado oil or nonstick cooking spray.

4. Place salmon skin side down on baking sheet. Pour/brush marinade over the top of the salmon.

5. For every inch of thickness, bake for 15 minutes. My salmon is usually perfect around 18-20 minutes. Flake salmon with a fork and serve. As a rule of thumb, it's best to undercook rather than overcook your salmon so that it doesn't dry out.

Nutrition Facts
Servings: **4**
Calories Per Serving: **200**
Macros:
Protein: 22g
Total Carbs: 0g
Fat: 13g

RyFit Tip:
I absolutely love cooking salmon in the oven so that it's moist, flavorful and stays together well. This is exactly how I bake it so it comes out perfectly every time.

Moroccan Spiced Salmon

Short on time? Try this delicious slow cooker recipe. The anti-inflammatory spice blend is savory, a bit sweet, and has the distinctive flavors of Morocco. You can customize the heat by adding more of less cayenne pepper.

Ingredients

4 x 6 oz ..... salmon fillets	3/4 tsp ...... salt
2 tbsp .... lemon juice, fresh squeezed	1/2 tsp ...... coriander, ground
2 tbsp .... olive oil	1/4 tsp ...... turmeric
1 tbsp .... paprika	1/4 tsp ...... cayenne pepper
1 tsp .... cumin	1/2 cup ...... cilantro, chopped to garnish

Preparation

1. Place all of the marinade ingredients into a large marinating bowl, then place the salmon in the bowl, making sure that the marinade coats both sides of the fish.

2. Cover and refrigerate for 4 to 6 hours.

3. Add 2 tbsp of water to a slow cooker or Crock-Pot, add fish, cover and cook for 1.5 to 2 hours on low. It can also be baked in the oven. When done let sit, uncovered, for five minutes before serving. Garnish each portion with cilantro.

Nutrition Facts
Servings: **4**
Calories Per Serving: **410**
Macros:
Protein: 38g
Total Carbs: 1.5g
Fat: 28g

RyFit Tip:
You can also cook this salmon in the oven with the same method as outlined in the Lemon Garlic Sweet Salmon recipe on the previous page.

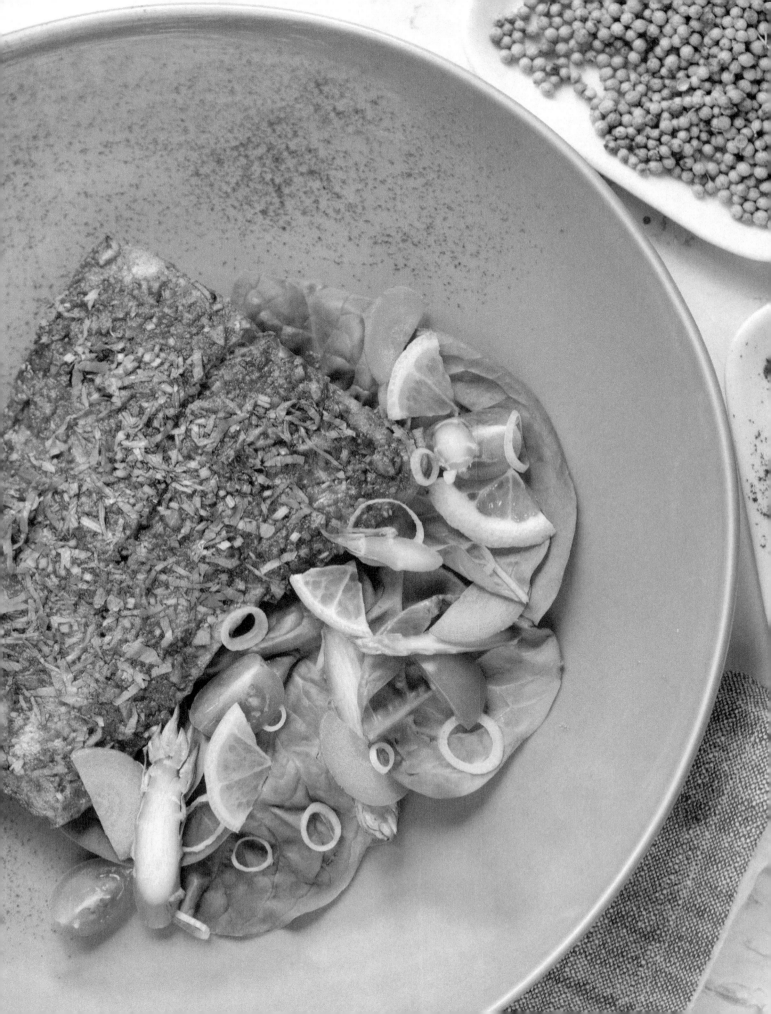

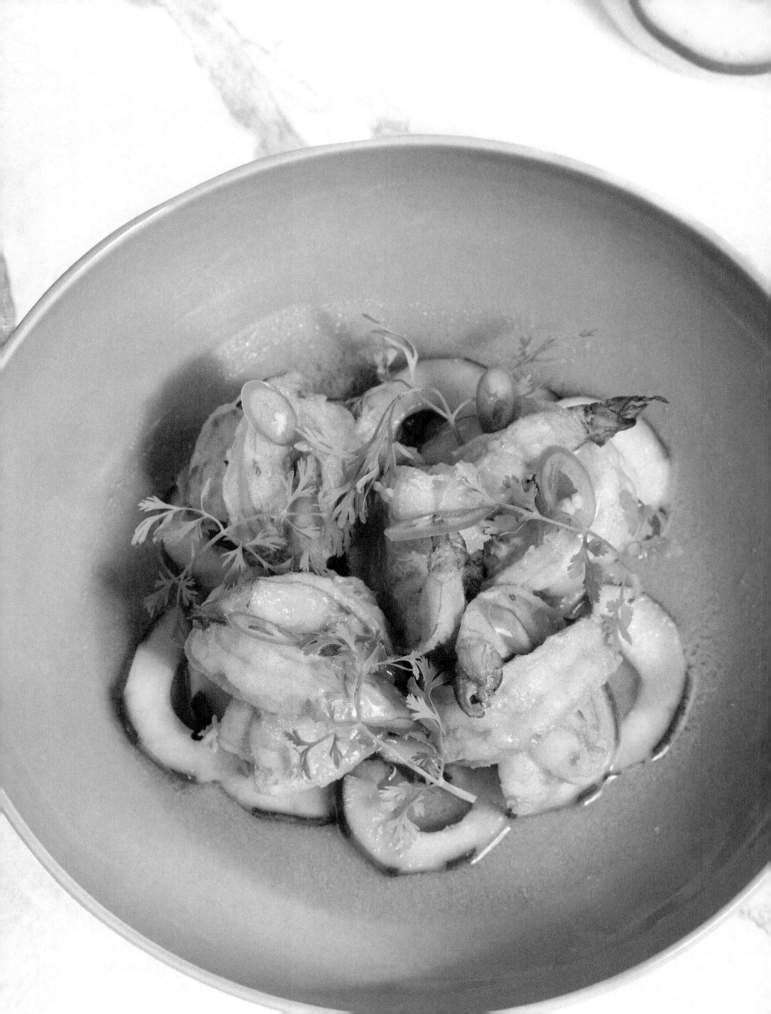

Green Curried Shrimp

A perfect combo of sweet, spicy and savory! I learned this recipe at cooking school in Chang Mai, Thailand and it's my favorite Thai recipe on the planet. I modified the fats to make it healthier and more flavorable. This is a great flavor for all your proteins and you'll want to compliment it with my coconut rice to make a complete meal.

Ingredients

2 tbsp .... olive oil

2 tbsp .... green curry paste

1 lb.......... shrimp, jumbo, shelled and deveined

4 .... kaffir lime leaves, torn

1............. lemongrass stalk

1 cup .... unsweetened coconut milk

2 tbsp .... fish sauce

1/2 .... cucumber, seeded and cut into thin strips

15 .... basil, fresh, leaves

4 .... green chillies, sliced to garnish
*optional

Preparation

1. Heat olive oil in a frying pan and add the curry paste fry until fragrant.

2. Toss in the shrimp, kaffir lime leaves and lemon grass (chop lemon grass for added flavor).

3. Fry for 1-2 minutes until prawns are pink.

4. Stir in the coconut milk and bring to a gentle boil, reduce to a simmer; stirring occasionally, for approximately 5 minutes.

5. Stir in the fish sauce, cucumber and basil. Serve and sprinkle with green chillies to garnish.

Nutrition Facts
Servings: **4**
Calories Per Serving: **168**
Macros:
Protein: 16g
Total Carbs: 2g (1g Fiber)
Fat: 8g

Teriyaki Grilled Salmon Salad

This grilled teriyaki salmon recipe has the perfect balance of sweet and smoky flavor. The garlic and coconut aminos in the teriyaki marinade make this salmon salad uniquely delicious.

Ingredients

Marinade

1 cup	orange juice, fresh squeezed
1/2 cup	coconut aminos
2 tbsp	rice vinegar
3 tbsp	monk fruit sweetener
1 tsp	garlic, minced
2 tsp	ginger root, minced

Salad

1 lb	salmon filets
1/2 cup	green onions, chopped, include bulb and some green
4 cups	Chinese cabbage, raw, shredded
1/2 cup	sweet red pepper, chopped
1/2 cup	shredded carrots

Preparation

1. In a small bowl mix together orange juice, coconut aminos, vinegar, monk fruit sweetener, garlic and ginger. Stir in the onion. Set aside ½ cup of the mixture.

2. Place salmon fillets (approximately 4) in a shallow dish and pour over the remaining marinade, turning to coat the whole fillet. Refrigerate for 30 minutes.

3. Make the salad by combining the cabbage, red pepper and carrots. Cover and chill.

4. Preheat the grill and grill at medium heat until done (approximately 10 minutes per inch of thickness).

5. Grill at medium heat until done, approximately 10 minutes per inch of thickness

6. Toss the reserved marinade with the prepared salad and top each serving with a piece of grilled salmon.

Nutrition Facts
Servings: **4**
Calories Per Serving: **299**
Macros:
Protein: 28g
Total Carbs: 11g
Fat: 10g

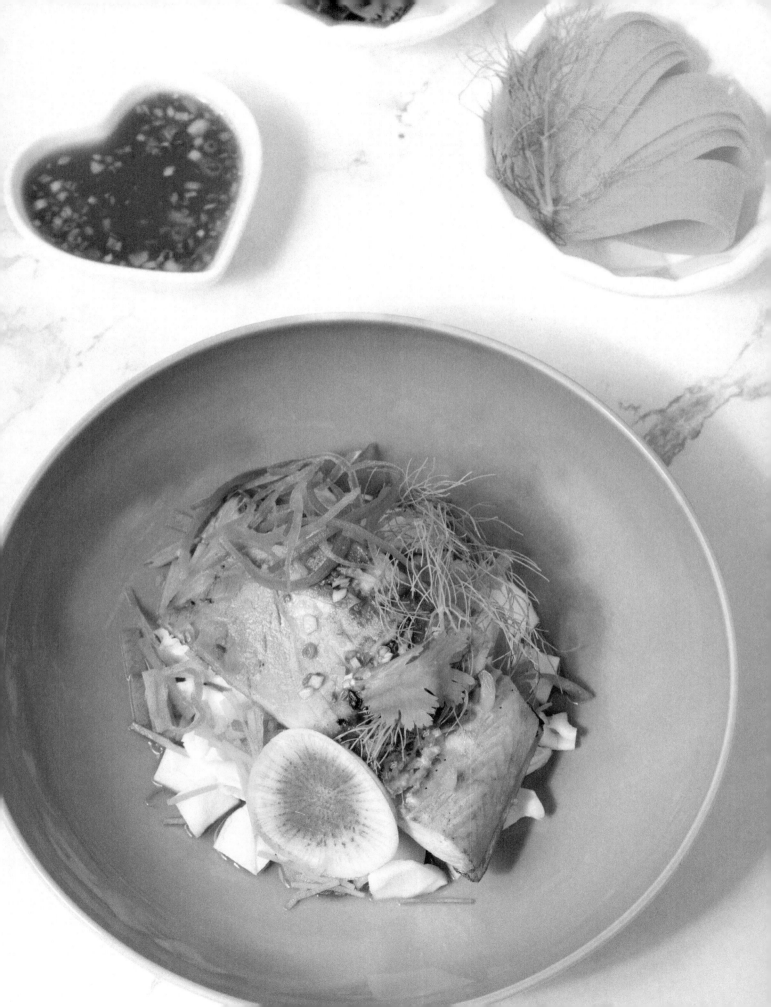

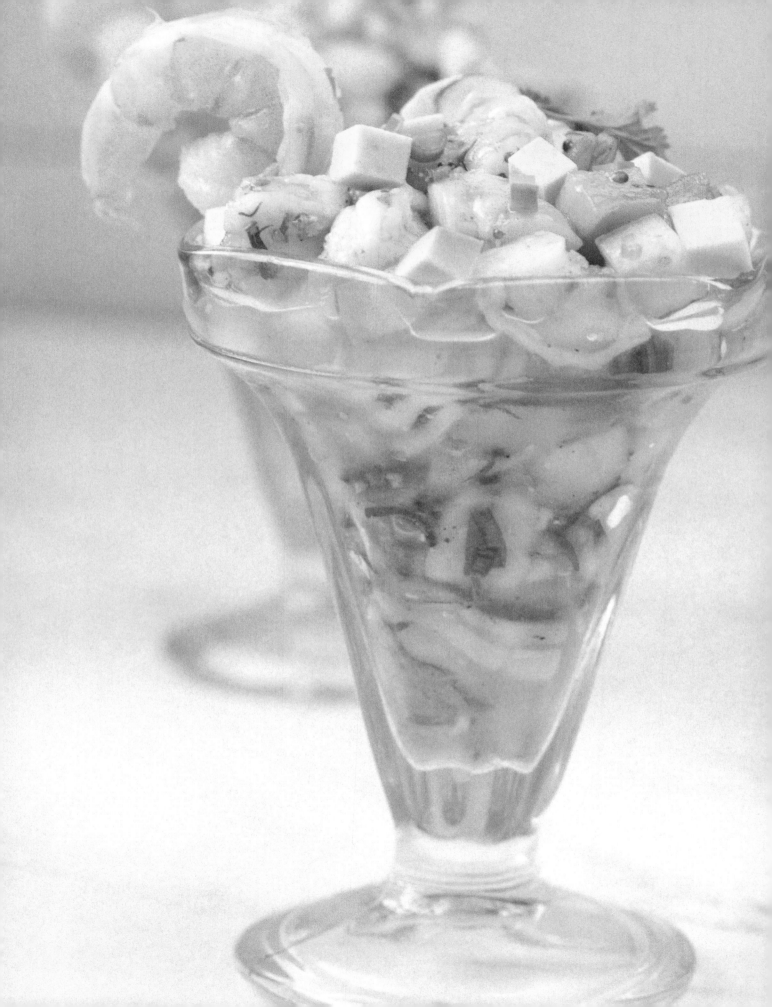

Mango Shrimp Cups

These protein packed cups are 'shrimply Irresistible' and one of my favorite light lunches - so fresh and delicious and no baking required. The combination of fresh mango with lime, cucumbers, avocado, tomatoes and onions is refreshing and satisfying. A perfect choice for a protein-packed starter or light meal - I promise you'll love them!

Ingredients

Dressing

- 2 tbsp .... olive oil
- 2 tbsp .... lime juice, freshly squeezed
- 1/2 tsp ...... monk fruit sweetener
- 1 tsp .... dijon mustard
- 1/2 tsp ...... lime zest, grated
- 1/4 tsp ...... salt & pepper
- 1/8 tsp....... cumin, ground
- 1/8 tsp ...... chili powder, ground

Salad

- 1 lb........... shrimp, large, chopped, cooked
  (don't use baby shrimp)
- 2.............. mangos, medium, cubed
- 1.............. avocado, large, cubed
- 1 cup .... English cucumbers, peeled, diced
- 1 cup .... grape tomatoes, quartered
- 2/3 cup ..... green onions, chopped
- 1/4cup ...... cilantro, chopped, fresh

Preparation

1. Whisk together all dressing ingredients in a small bowl. Refrigerate until ready to use.

2. Combine all salad ingredients in a large bowl. Mix gently to avoid mashing the avocados. Give dressing a quick whisk and add to salad. Mix gently until salad is coated with dressing. Add a bit more salt & pepper, if desired. Divide salad among small cups, and serve with small spoons.

Nutrition Facts
Servings: **8**
Calories Per Serving: **167**
Macros:
Protein: 13g
Total Carbs: 13g (3g Fiber)
Fat: 8g

RyFit Tip:
Try fresh peaches for mango when they're in season.

Fit Fish Tacos

I've become a loyal taco fan since moving to Mexico. However, often they're made with unhealthy battered and fried fish and use tortillas made with inflammatory ingredients. Here's my lighter and healthier version that is ABS-olutely freaking 'fish delish'.

Ingredients

Filling

1	avocado
1/2 cup	black beans
1/2 cup	cabbage slaw
8 oz	white fish (Mahi Mahi or Red Snapper are my favs!)
4 tbsp	salsa
2 tbsp	guacamole
6	tortillas, small, whole wheat, non GMO corn, keto tortilla or make your own gluten free protein tortillas (recipe on page 241)

Marinade

2 tbsp	olive oil
1	lime, juiced
1 tbsp	chili powder
1 tsp	paprika
1 tsp	garlic powder
1	jalapeño, chopped *optional
1/2 cup	cilantro, fresh, chopped

Preparation

1. Mix all marinade ingredients together and pour over the fish. Let marinate for 20 minutes.

2. Heat a grill or non-stick pan to medium. Remove fish from marinade and cook for 4-5 minutes; until fish is flakey and cooked through, but still soft.

3. Distribute fish evenly into 2 servings and place in your tortillas. Add the rest of the filling ingredients, hot sauce (if you like it spicy) and enjoy!

Nutrition Facts
*calculated using 3 gluten free protein tortillas
Servings: **2**
Calories Per Serving: **410**
Macros:
Protein: 36g
Total Carbs: 37g (5g Fiber)
Fat: 17g

RyFit Tip:

Looking for a lighter option? Remove the beans and add more veggies. Use my home-made gluten free protein tortillas to boost your protein and fiber!

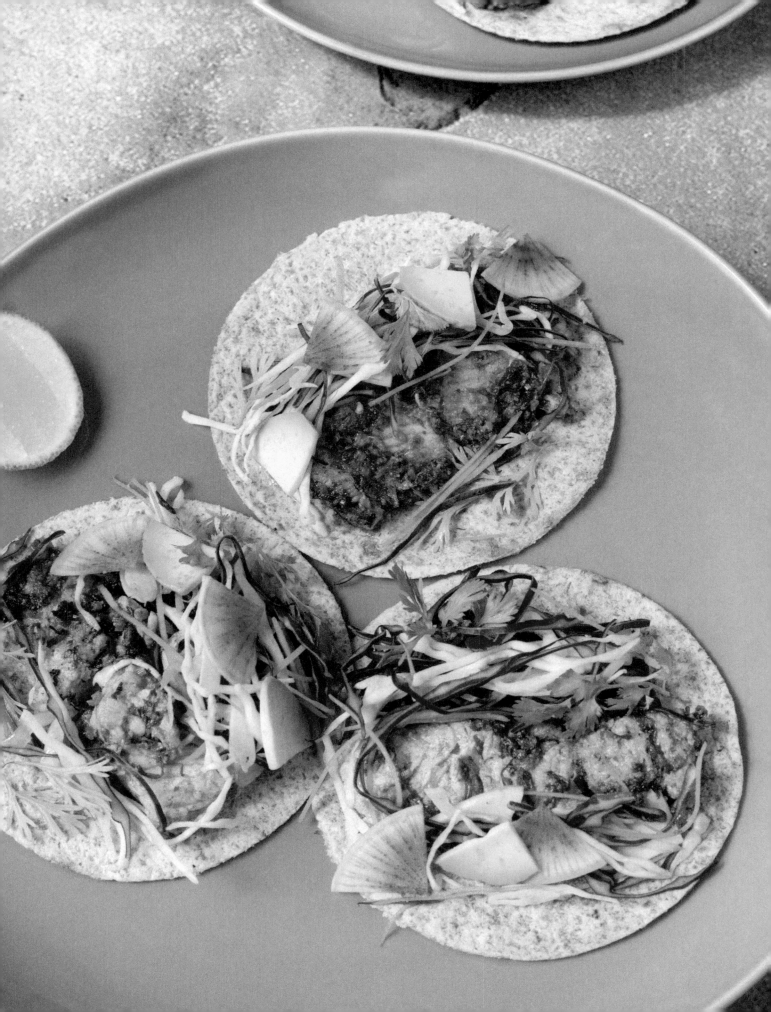

Keep it Tight Tuna Salad

A simple way to 'sex up' raw or leftover vegetables without adding excess calories in under 5 minutes. You can substitute chicken for tuna. In a pinch for time? Pull apart a roast chicken from the grocery store and you've got a meal.

Ingredients

Sauce

1 tbsp .... avocado or olive oil mayonnaise

4 tbsp....... Greek yogurt, plain, fat free

1.............. lime to taste

1/4 tsp ...... salt & pepper

1 tbsp .... mustard

Base

4 cups....... broccoli, carrots, beets, celery, raw or your leftover vegetables

2 x 6 oz ..... albacore wild tuna, canned

Preparation

Combine sauce ingredients together in a bowl and fold into into protein & veggies and voila - it's like an entirely new meal! I enjoy this on it's own as a light meal, on top of rice cakes or as a filling inside of a wrap.

Nutrition Facts
Servings: **2**
Calories Per Serving: **298**
Macros:
Protein: 33g
Total Carbs: 4g
Fat: 9g

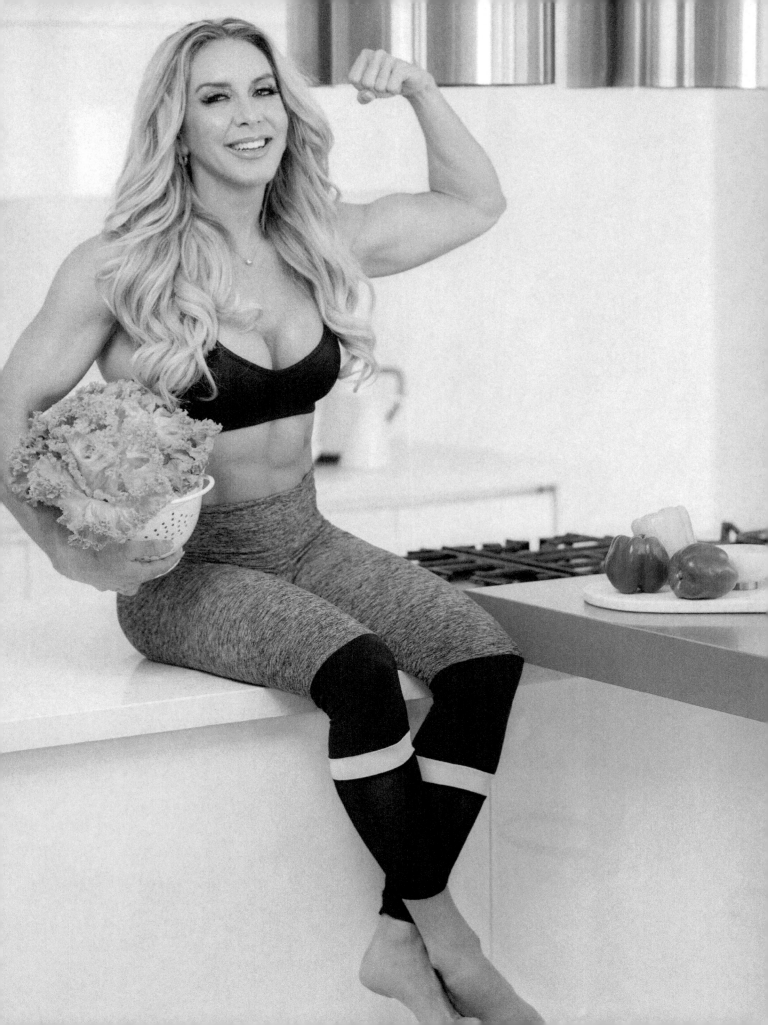

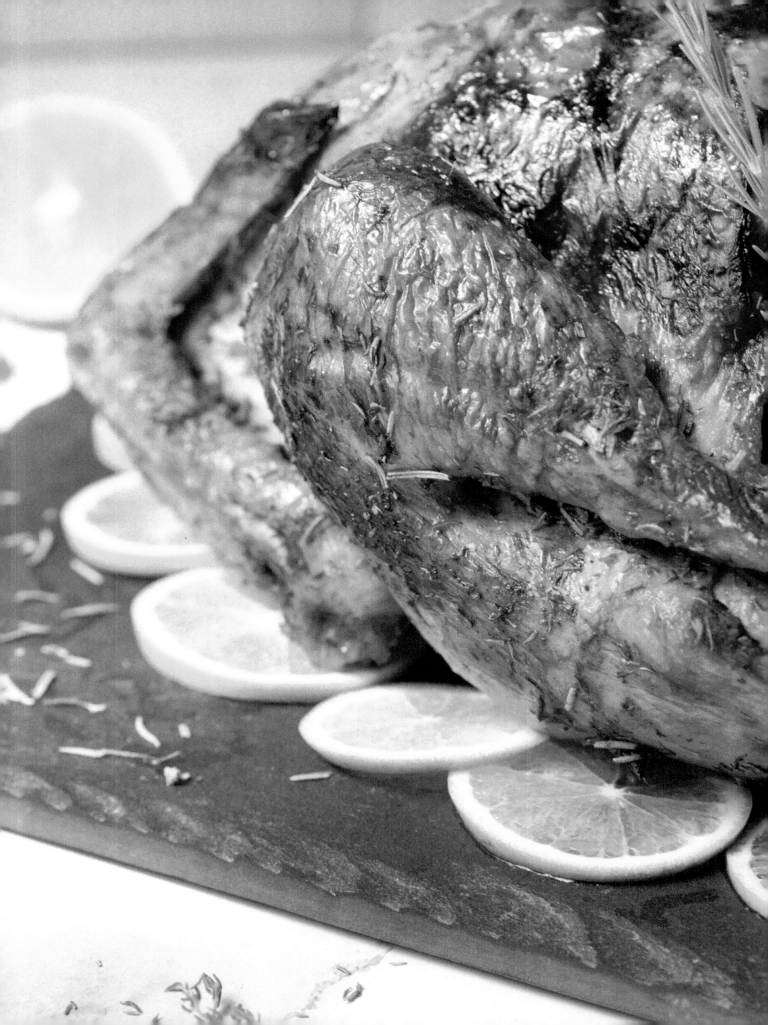

POUTLRY

From skewered breasts to roasted thighs, you'll be more than satisfied with these flavorful and juicy poultry recipes. Pair these proteins with a colorful side dish when planning your weekly meals to create nutritious, balanced meals. Opt for pasture-raised when possible for the cleanest cuts.

Spicy SouthWest Power Bowl

Power bowls are so fun for family meals because you can switch up the veggies and toppings to suit each palate, giving kids control to build their own bowls. Transform your leftovers into a perfect post-workout meal or a quick and easy dinner for busy weeknights.

Ingredients

4 oz .... chicken breast, grilled or baked and sliced	1/4 .... Roma tomato, chopped
1/2 cup ..... black beans, cooked	1 tsp .... olive oil
1/2 cup ...... brown rice, cooked	1/2 tsp ...... paprika
1/4 cup ..... corn, roasted	1/2 tsp ...... garlic powder
1/4 .... onion, chopped	1/2 tsp ...... oregano
	1/4 .... avocado

Preparation

1. Grill or bake chicken and season with paprika, garlic powder, oregano, salt & pepper.

2. In a non-stick pan sauté onion with olive oil until translucent.

3. Add black beans, corn, tomato and continue to cook for 5 more minutes.

4. Place warm bean mixture on top of rice in bowl. Top with chicken, avocado and salsa (optional).

Nutrition Facts
Servings: **3**
Calories Per Serving: **335**
Macros:
Protein: 18g
Total Carbs: 47g (7g Fiber)
Fat: 9g

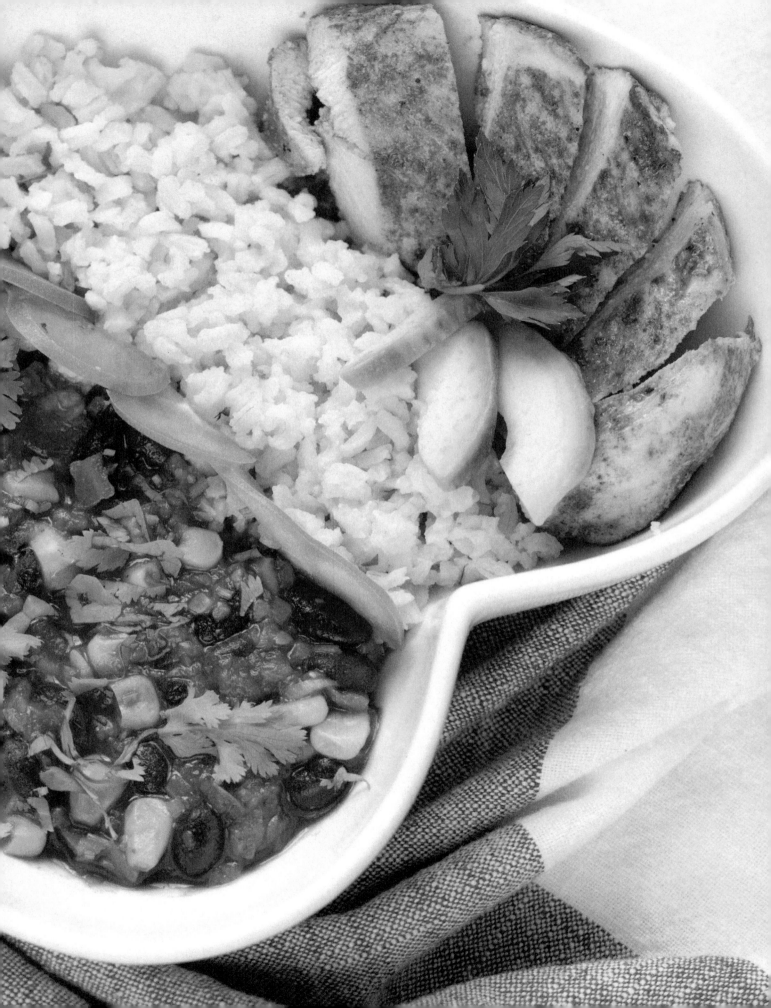

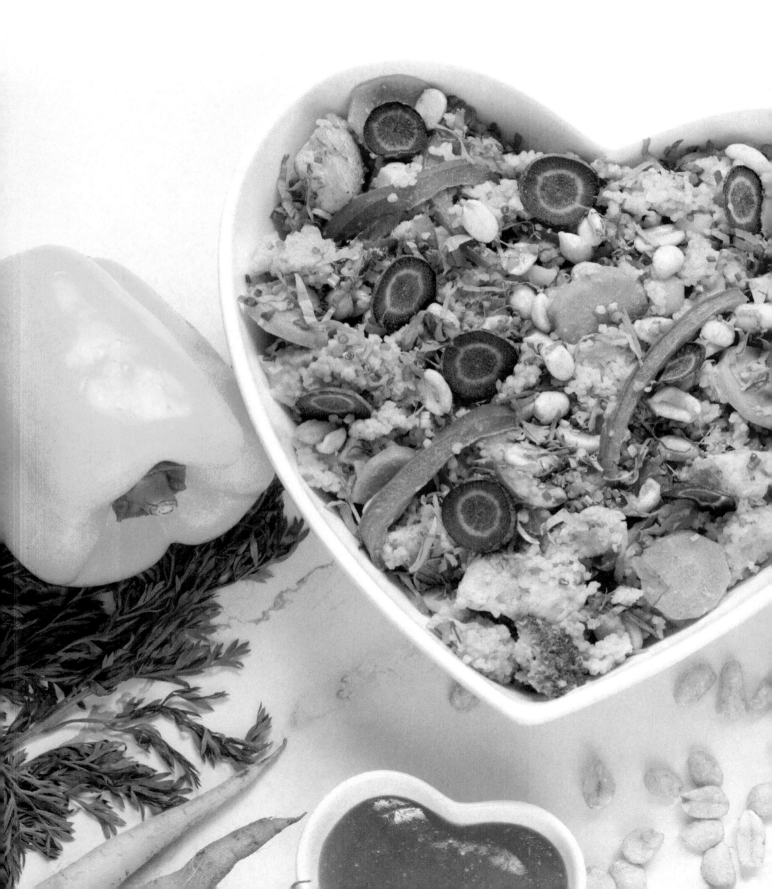

Thai Peanut Chicken Couscous

This meal is SO freaking satisfying AND simple to whip up! All made in one single pan, it's loaded with protein, rich and creamy flavor and colorful veggies. Substitute quinoa for couscous to make this gluten-free and slightly reduce the glycemic load - a perfect pre-workout meal or lunch.

Ingredients

For the peanut couscous:

1 cup	....	israeli pearl couscous
3	....	garlic cloves, minced
2 cup	....	unsweetened coconut milk
3/4 cup	.....	chicken broth, low sodium
		(or substitute water)
1/2 cup	.....	peanut butter, natural, creamy
3 tbsp	......	coconut aminos
1 tbsp	....	ginger, freshly grated
1 tbsp	....	chili paste or sriracha

For the chicken:

1 tbsp	....	avocado oil or olive oil
1 lb	....	chicken breast, boneless, skinless, cubed
1/4 tsp	......	salt & pepper

Add ins:

2	....	carrots, large, thinly sliced
3 cup	....	broccoli florets
1	....	red bell pepper, thinly sliced

To garnish:

green onion (green part only), **diced, fresh chopped cilantro, roasted peanuts or hot sauce.**

Preparation

1. Brown your chicken so it's golden brown. No need to cook it all the way through.

2. Now make the peanut sauce. In the same skillet you'll stir together the coconut milk, broth, peanut butter, coconut aminos, ginger & chili paste. Super simple as it's all in one skillet!

3. Once your peanut sauce is smooth you'll stir in the couscous and veggies.

4. Add your chicken and bring to a simmer, then reduce the heat and cover the pan for 15 minutes.

5. Let it thicken for a few minutes uncovered.

6. Top with your fav garnishes, extra hot sauce (if you desire), and serve!

Note: the consistency is a bit more mushy with the quinoa.

Nutrition Facts
Servings: **6**
Calories Per Serving: **415**
Macros:
Protein: 29g
Total Carbs: 34g (5g Fiber)
Fat: 18.5g

Maple Mushroom Chicken

Theres something about maple and mushroom that I love. It's sweet, savory and satisfying. If you like a little sweet with your meat but don't want the added sugar then you're going to love this dish!

Ingredients

10 oz .... chicken breast

1 tbsp .... sesame seed oil

1 tbsp .... olive oil

2 .... garlic cloves, fresh, minced and peeled

1/4 .... red onion, diced and peeled

3 cups ...... mushroom

1/4 cup ..... coconut aminos

1/4 .... sugar free maple syrup

1/4 tsp ...... salt

Preparation

1. Brown your chicken in olive oil.

2. Remove from frying pan and add the sesame oil, garlic and onion to the same flying pan. Simmer on low/medium heat for 3 minutes.

3. Add mushrooms (use as many different varieties of mushrooms as possible) and coconut aminos. Cook covered until mushrooms are soft. Add the maple syrup and cubed chicken.

4. Cook for 2 more minutes on low heat. Serve over a bed of my coconut basmati rice or with sweet potatoes. And, of course, enjoy a colorful side salad or veggies!

Nutrition Facts
Servings: **4**
Calories Per Serving: **172**
Macros:
Protein: 17g
Total Carbs: 5.9g
Fat: 5g

RyFit Tip:
This recipe is one of my favorites for adding flavor without heavy calories to any protein dish. Swap the chicken for tofu, beef or turkey, add asparagus for a nutritional boost and use chicken thighs for more tender, flavorful chicken for just a bit more calories from fat.

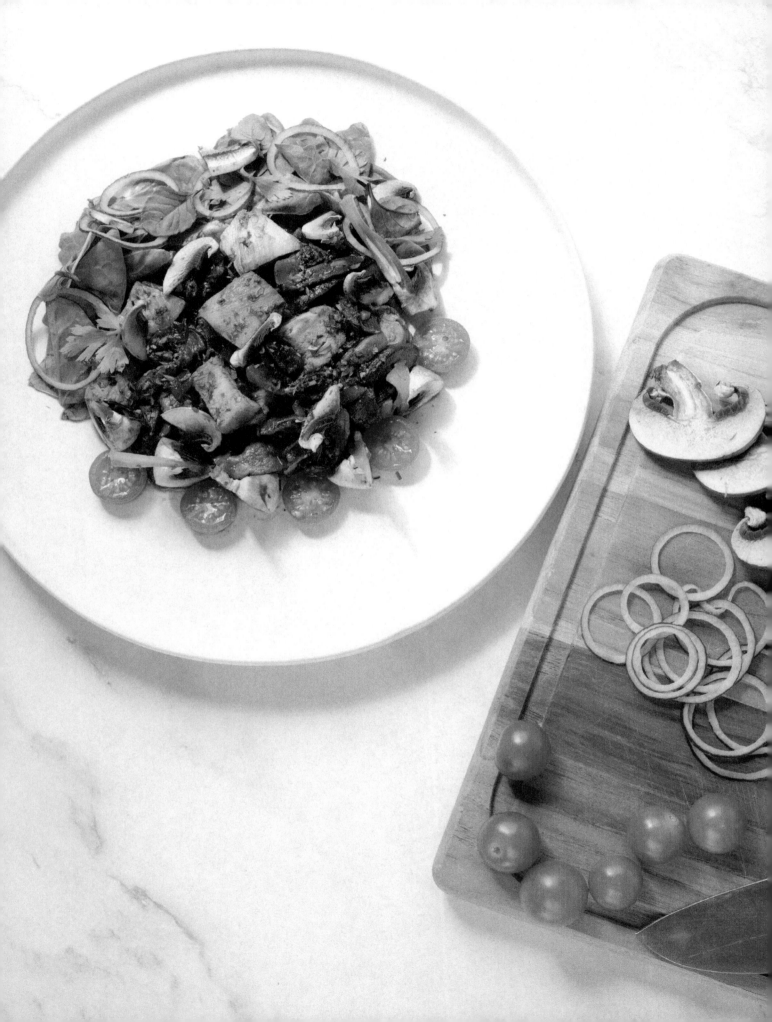

Healthy Chicken Nuggets

My Healthy Baked Chicken Nuggets are made with strips of chicken breasts coated in oats, Italian seasoning, adaptogenic mushroom powder and hormone-balancing maca and then baked until golden. An easy chicken recipe that your entire family will love.

Ingredients

2 x 5 oz...... skinless chicken breasts, raw

1/4 cup ..... egg whites

1/4 cup ..... oatmeal, small flake

1/4 cup ..... sliced almonds, crushed

1 tbsp .... Italian seasoning

1 tbsp .... maca

1 tbsp .... mushroom powder *optional

1 tsp .... salt

1 tsp .... pepper

Preparation

1. Preheat oven to 350 F. Coat a baking sheet with cooking spray.

2. Cut chicken into strips. Pour egg whites over chicken strips to coat.

3. In a blender, combine oats, maca, almonds and seasonings. Place chicken strips in a marinating bowl with the oat mixture and shake. You can add a dash of parmesan cheese if you want as well.

4. Remove chicken from bowl and place on baking sheet. Bake for 20 minutes, until chicken is cooked through.

5. You'll love them with my yogurt dip on page 309.

Nutrition Facts
Servings: **2**
Calories Per Serving: **270**
Macros:
Protein: 40g
Total Carbs: 11g (3g Fiber)
Fat: 8g

Slow Cooker Balsamic Chicken

This is a damn delicious way to enjoy chicken. Let the crockpot do all of the work - it's the easiest dish of all time. Simply throw everything in with a 5 minute prep!

Ingredients

5 x 5 oz ..... skinless chicken breast, raw

1/2 cup ..... balsamic vinegar

1 .... onion, small

1 tsp .... garlic, minced

1 tbsp .... basil, fresh *preferred over dry

1/4 tsp ...... salt

1/4 tsp ...... pepper

2 tbsp ...... olive oil

Preparation

1. Coat bottom of the crock pot with 2 tbsp of olive oil, add chicken breast on top.

2. Top the chicken with pepper, salt, minced garlic, chopped onion, and a sprinkle of basil.

Pour ½ cup of balsamic vinegar on top and let chicken cook for 4 hours on high (or 8 hours on low).

Nutrition Facts

Servings: **5**

Calories Per Serving: **288**

Macros:

Protein: 55g

Total Carbs: 6g (1g Fiber)

Fat: 3g

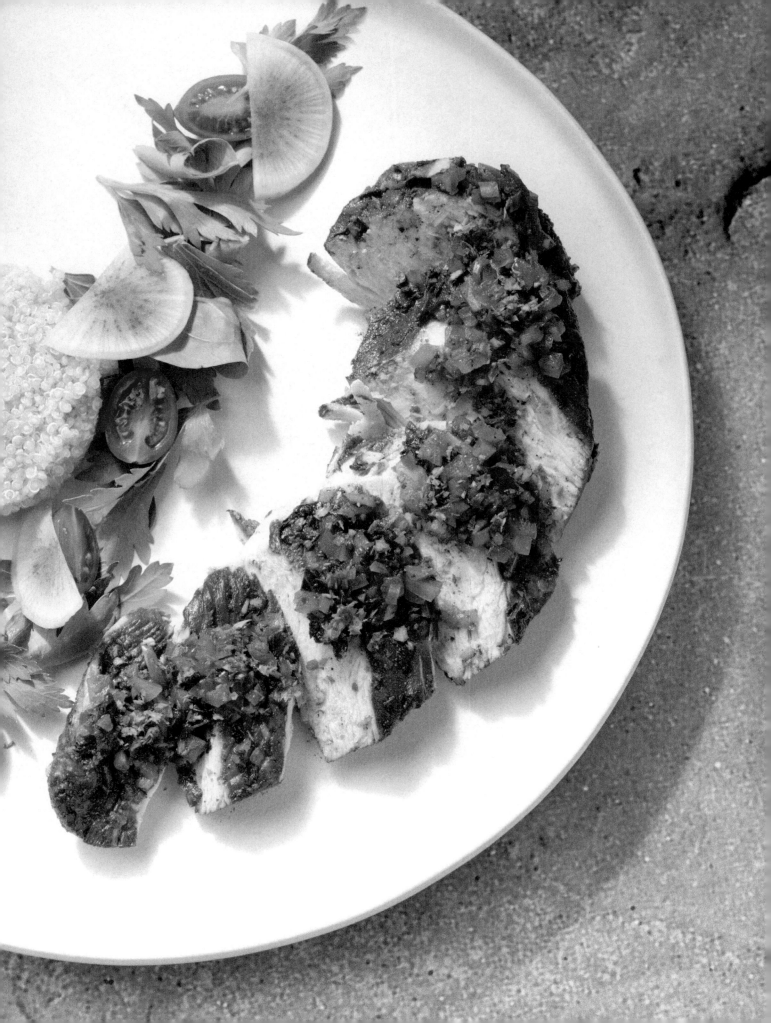

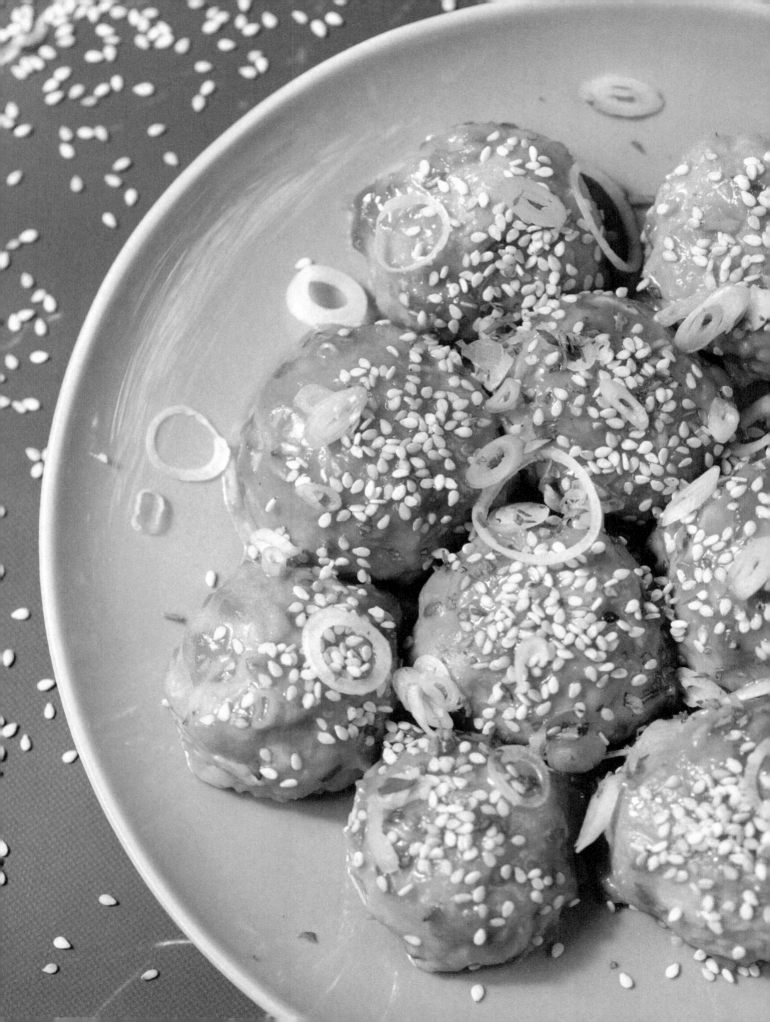

Sweet & Spicy Turkey Meatballs

Perfect as an appetizer or served over rice for an entrée, these sweet and spicy turkey meatballs prove that healthy foods can also be flavorful! Added plant based fatty acids and digestion boosting ginger make this turkey next-level. This is an awesome recipe with chicken as well.

Ingredients

Balls

2 lbs (1kg) ..	turkey, ground
1/2 cup	gluten free oats
2 tbsp	hoisin sauce
1	egg
2 tsp	garlic, minced
1 tbsp	flax seed
1 tsp	ginger, fresh
1 tsp	sesame oil, dark
1/2 tsp	salt

Glaze

1 cup	apricot jam, no-sugar added
1/4 cup	coconut aminos
1 tbsp	lime, fresh juiced
2 tsp	garlic, minced
2 tsp	ginger, grated, fresh
1/2 tsp	sesame oil, dark
1 tbsp	sriracha hot sauce *optional

Preparation

1. Preheat oven to 400F. Combine all the meat ball ingredients in a bowl and mix. Form them into balls with your hands (wet hands if they're sticky!) and place on non-stick baking sheet. Bake in preheated oven for 15-18 min. Flip once to brown all sides.

2. Glaze is easy - whisk together all ingredients in deep non-stick skillet. Cook over medium heat and when jam has melted and its bubbling add meat balls and mix gently to sauce them up. Garnish with some sesame seeds and green onions

---

Nutrition Facts

Servings: **8**

Calories Per Serving: **280**

Macros:
Protein: 33g
Total Carbs: 11g (3g Fiber)
Fat: 14g

RyFit Tip:
Want to make this carb free? Substitute 1/4 cup coconut flour for the gluten free oats.

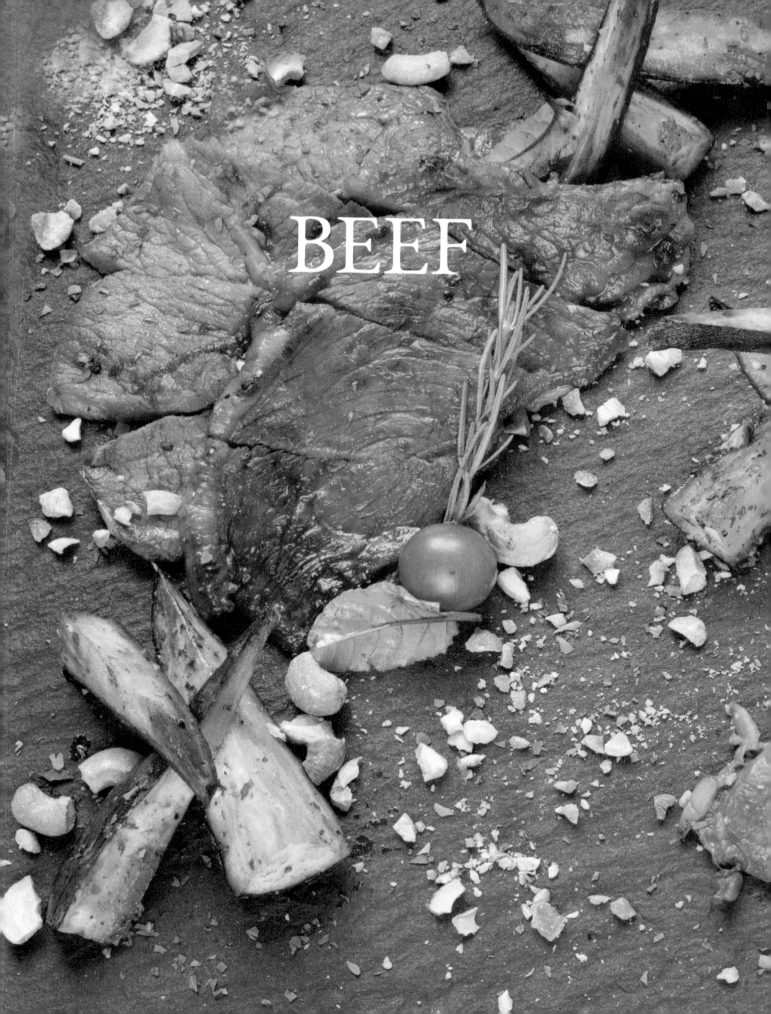

BEEF

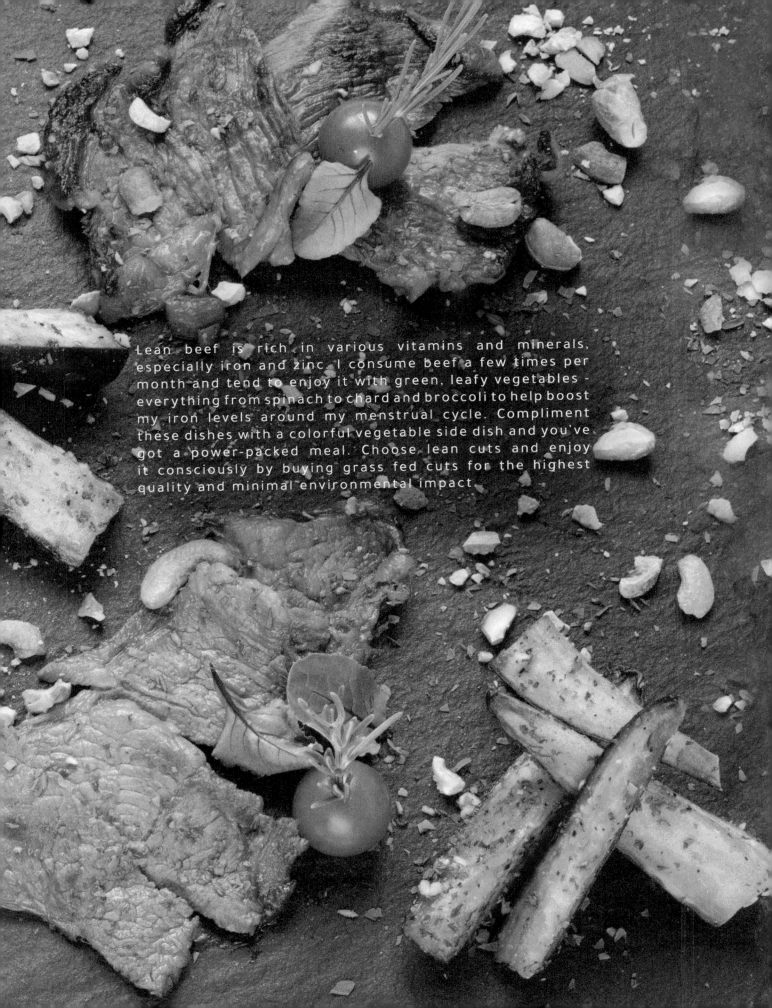

Lean beef is rich in various vitamins and minerals, especially iron and zinc. I consume beef a few times per month and tend to enjoy it with green, leafy vegetables - everything from spinach to chard and broccoli to help boost my iron levels around my menstrual cycle. Compliment these dishes with a colorful vegetable side dish and you've got a power-packed meal. Choose lean cuts and enjoy it consciously by buying grass fed cuts for the highest quality and minimal environmental impact.

Lean and Mean Meat Balls

Baked meat balls are the best and these are just so super simple to whip up - in no time you'll have a whole pan of meatballs that are cooked through and ready to eat either by themselves, or thrown in sauce over lentil pasta, whole grain rice or vegetables. No more cooking meatballs in batches or standing by the stovetop! Plus, these are great to have your kids help with!

Ingredients

1 lb........... ground beef, extra lean

1 tbsp .... parsley, minced

1/2 cup...... onion, finely chopped

1/2 tsp ...... salt

1/2 tsp ...... pepper

1.............. whole egg

1 tbsp .... olive oil

1/4 cup...... cheese, mozzarella, organic

Preparation

1. Combine all ingredients in a bowl and hand stir until fully combined. Cheese is optional but will add moisture and flavor.

2. Form into balls. Cook either in the oven at 375F for 20 minutes or in a frying pan sprayed with olive oil on medium-high heat until they're brown and cooked through.

Nutrition Facts
Servings: **4**
Calories Per Serving: **255**
Macros:
Protein: 31g
Total Carbs: 1.7g (.5g Fiber)
Fat: 9.5g

RyFit Tip:
Add a a few teaspoons of superfood powders like mushrooms, moringa or maca to boost the health benefits.

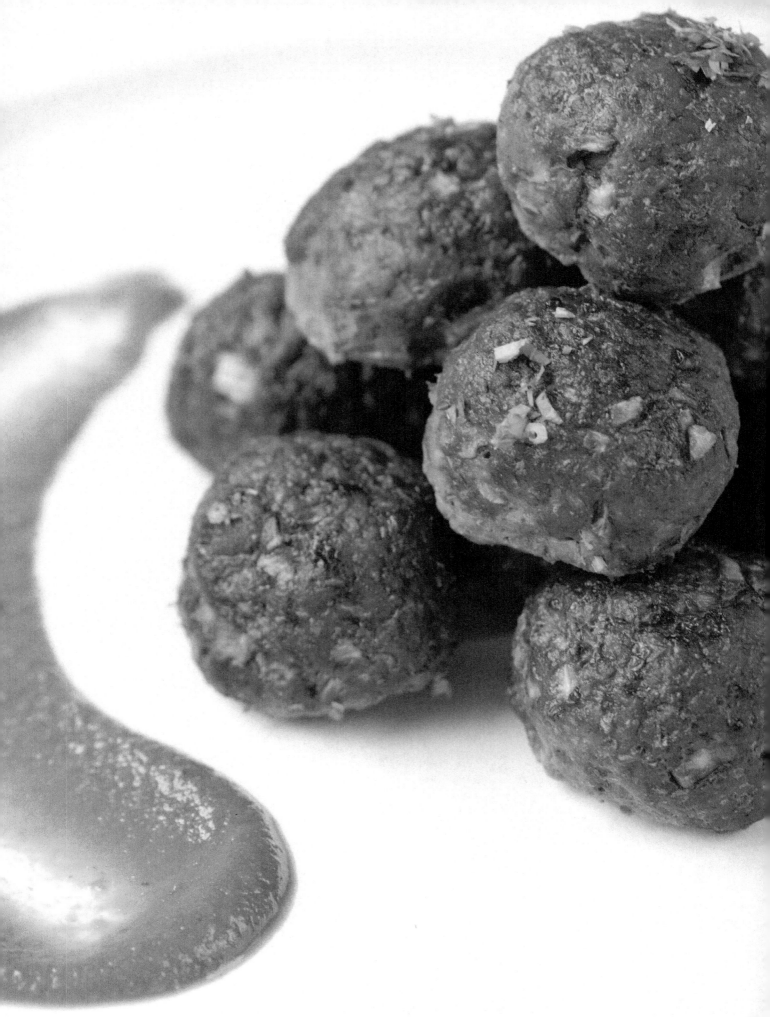

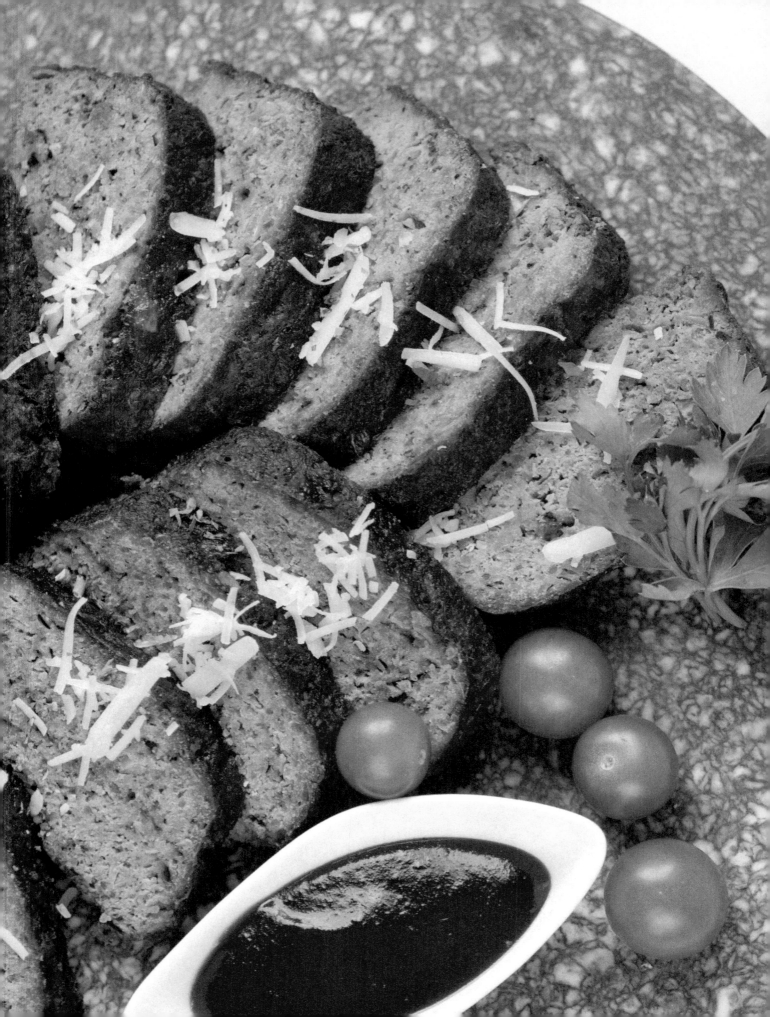

Maca Meatloaf

When I think of meatloaf I think of my childhood in Canada - a warm, hearty meal on a cold winter night. This is my heathy twist on my Mom's traditional meatloaf. Quinoa combined with basil, parsley, garlic and hormone-supporting maca make this a favorable, healthy and nutritious meal. Quick to whip up and makes great left overs!

Ingredients

2 lbs	ground beef, extra-lean
1 cup	quinoa, cooked
1/3 cup......	Parmesan cheese, freshly grated
1/2 cup......	barbecue sauce, no sugar added
1..............	whole egg
1 tbsp	maca

1/4 cup......	parsley, fresh, chopped
1/4 cup......	onions, finely minced or grated
2 tsp........	garlic, minced
1 tsp	basil, dried
1/2 tsp	pepper

Preparation

1. In a large bowl, combine all ingredients except 1/4 cup barbecue sauce. Mix well using your hands. Form mixture into 8 x 4-inch loaf pan with cooking spray (or line bottom of pan with foil for easy clean up!).

2. Cover top and sides of loaf with remaining 1/4 cup barbecue sauce. Bake at 350F for about 1 hour and 20 minutes, or until meatloaf is cooked through. Let meatloaf cool before serving for easier slicing.

Nutrition Facts
Servings: **6**
Calories Per Serving: **292**
Macros:
Protein: 34g
Total Carbs: 14g (1g Fiber)
Fat: 10g

Say goodbye to high calorie, unsatisfying and garbage-ingredient bottled dressings and hello to these fresh, protein-packed Greek yogurt dips. They're flavorful, thick, creamy, and long to be smeared on your healthy sandwich, dunked into with protein or veggies. Simply whip together the ingredients with a fork and enjoy! Each recipe makes approximately 4 servings.

Chili Yogurt Dip

Ingredients

1 cup	Greek yogurt, 0% plain
2 tbsp	lime juice, freshly squeezed
1 tsp.	monk fruit sweetener
1-4 tsp	chili powder
	(add to your taste preference)
1 tsp.	cumin, ground
¼ tsp.......	salt & pepper

Tzatziki Yogurt Dip

Ingredients

1 cup	Greek yogurt, 0% plain
3/4 cup	English cucumbers, peeled and finely diced
1 tbsp	lemon juice, fresh squeezed
1 tbsp	dill, minced, fresh
1 tbsp	monk fruit sweetener
1 tsp	garlic, minced
1/4 tsp	salt & pepper

Nutrition Facts
Servings: 4
Calories Per Serving: **25**
Macros:
Protein: 5g
Total Carbs: 3g
Fat: 1g

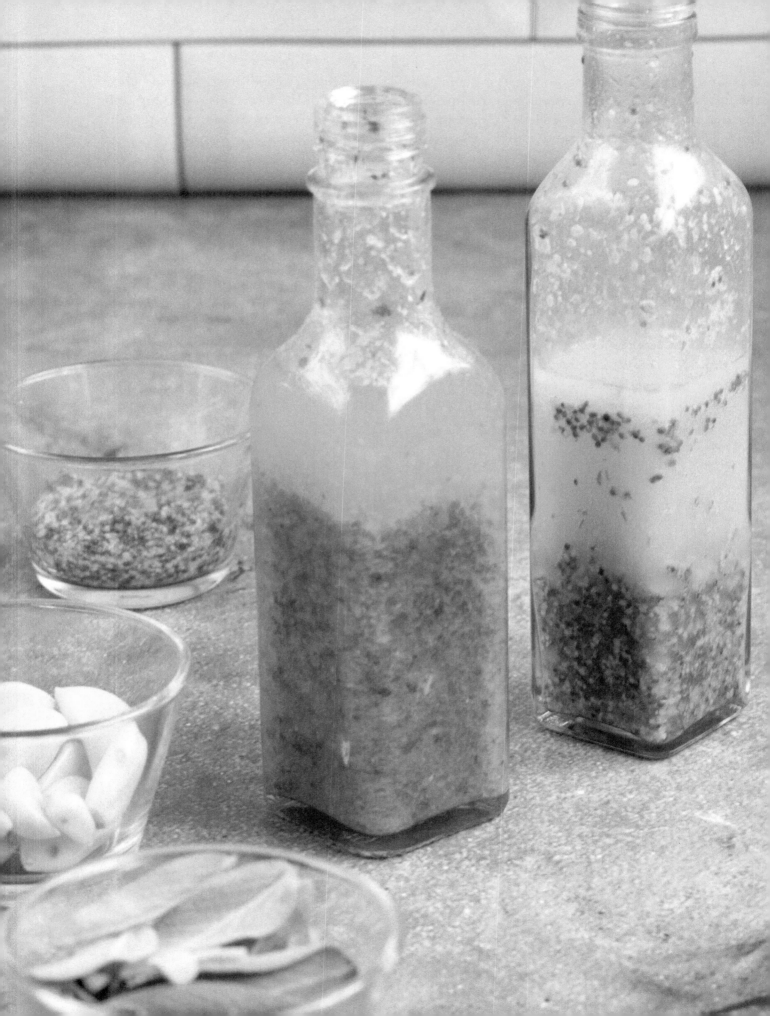

Ry's Homemade Herb Meat Marinades

Ingredients

Protein: Chicken
- garlic
- parsley
- onion
- basil

Protein: Fish
- ginger
- coriander
- dill
- cilantro
- fennel

Preparation

1. Combine a handful of each of the fresh herbs and items as outlined with 1 cup of olive oil. Blend in a food processor or blender and pour onto fresh meat to marinade at least 20 minutes before cooking. Store the excess in a bottle in your fridge and save it for your next meal prep! It'll last up to a month.

RyFit Tip:
Freeze your fresh meats pre-marinated.

Ghee Goodness White Fish Marinade

Ingredients

- 1/4 cup...... ghee, organic, grass-fed
- 1 tbsp........ lime, fresh squeezed
- 2 tbsp........ dijon mustard
- 2 tbsp........ parsley, fresh, grated

Nutrition Facts
Calories Per Serving: **400**
Macros:
Protein: .5g
Total Carbs: 0g
Fat: 46g

Preparation

1. Combine all ingredients in a marinating bowl. Blend with a fork and coat fish well for at least 2 hours. Remove from marinade and cook stove top or bake. A delicious marinade with healthy fats for white fish.

RyFit Tip:
Does a marinade add calories? Not much. A lot of the marinating liquid drips off the meat before it is consumed.
Enjoy!

Home-made High Intensity Herb Salad Dressing

This is my favorite home made salad dressing. Bursting with flavor, heart-healthy fat and fat-burning vinegar. When I eat in a restaurant I take a small portion of this with me to avoid restaurant dressings that can be loaded with poor quality vegetable oils and preservatives.

Ingredients

Base:
- 1/3 cup ...... olive oil
- 1/8 cup ...... balsamic vinegar
- 1/8 cup ...... malt vinegar

Fresh herbs to taste:
- 1 tbsp .... parsley
- 1 tbsp .... basil
- 1 tbsp .... ginger
- 1 tbsp .... coriander

Preparation

1. Combine and blend in a blender. Store in a sealed container in your fridge for up to one month.

Nutrition Facts (1 tbsp)
Servings: **7**
Calories Per Serving: **90**
Macros:
Protein: .5g
Total Carbs: .5g
Fat: 11g

Acai Dressing

Ingredients

1/3 cup......	olive oil
3 tbsp.......	apple cider vinegar
2 tbsp.......	dijon mustard
1 tsp.........	acai powder or 2 tbsp mulled berries
2 tbsp.......	sugar free maple syrup
1 whole.....	lemon, fresh squeezed
1/8 tsp......	salt & pepper

Nutrition Facts (1 tbsp)

Servings: **7**

Calories Per Serving: **95**

Macros:

Protein: .5g

Total Carbs: 2g

Fat: 7g

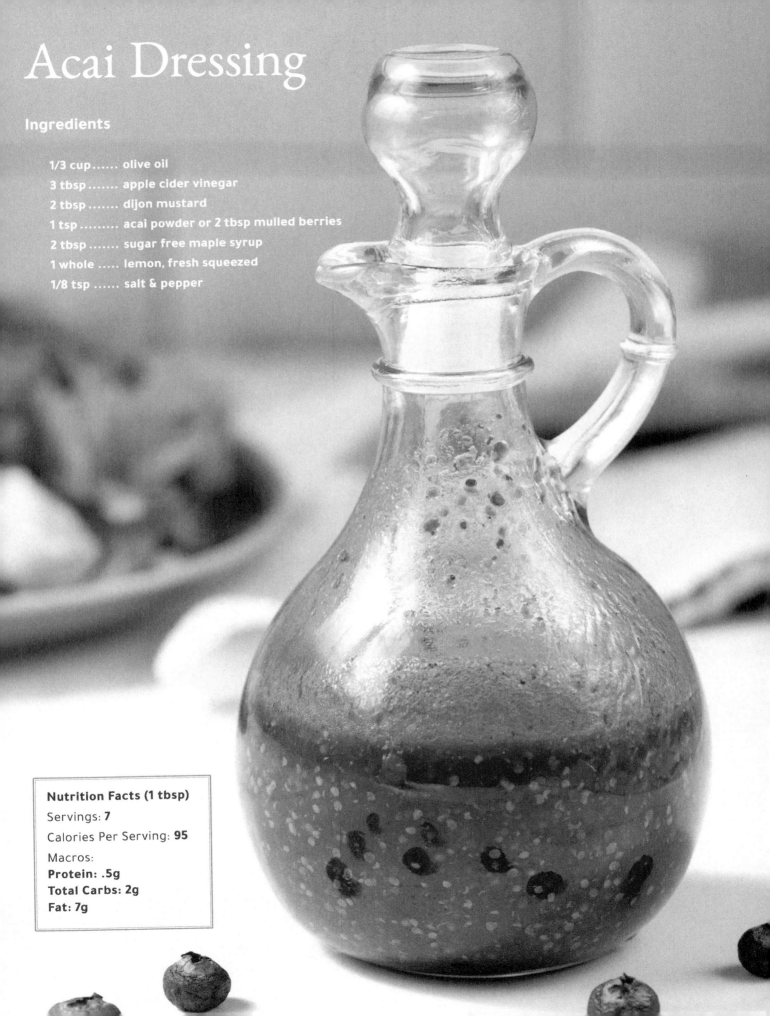

Japanese Dressing

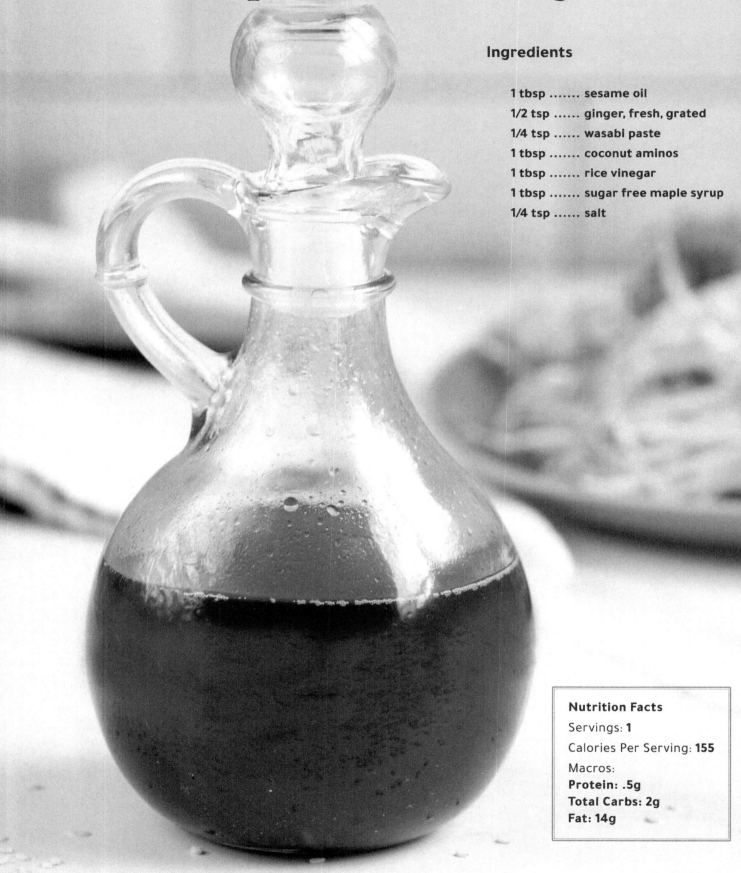

Ingredients

1 tbsp	sesame oil
1/2 tsp	ginger, fresh, grated
1/4 tsp	wasabi paste
1 tbsp	coconut aminos
1 tbsp	rice vinegar
1 tbsp	sugar free maple syrup
1/4 tsp	salt

Nutrition Facts

Servings: **1**

Calories Per Serving: **155**

Macros:

Protein: .5g

Total Carbs: 2g

Fat: 14g

Tahini Citrus Dressing

Ingredients

- 1/3 cup ...... tahini
- 1/3 cup ...... water
- 2 tbsp .... lemon juice
- 2 tbsp .... orange juice + pinch of zest
- 1 .... garlic clove, grated
- 2 tsp .... sugar free maple syrup
- 1/4 tsp ...... salt
- 1/2 tsp ...... chickpea miso paste or fish sauce
- 3/4 inch ..... ginger, fresh, grated

Nutrition Facts

Servings: **3**

Calories Per Serving: **100**

Macros:

Protein: 3g

Total Carbs: 1g

Fat: 8g

Ah-mazing Almond Butter Sauce

Ingredients

1/2 cup ...... almond butter

1/8 cup ...... tahini

1/4 cup ...... coconut aminos

2 tbsp .... lime juice

1 tsp .... ginger, grated

1 .... garlic clove, grated

1 tsp .... chile paste

1/4 cup ...... water

1 .... medjool date, pitted

Preparation

1. In a food processor, combine all ingredients and blend until smooth.
Transfer to a serving bowl to serve.
So satisfying and delicious!

Nutrition Facts

Servings: **7**

Calories Per Serving: **130**

Macros:
Protein: 12g
Total Carbs: 1g
Fat: 3g

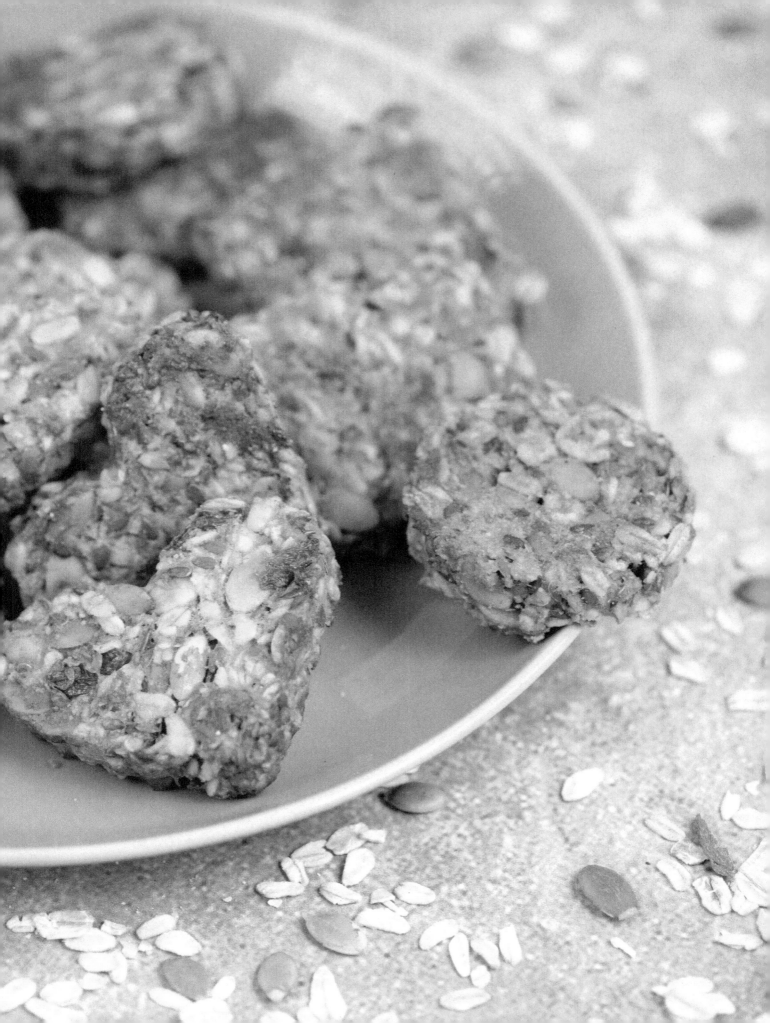

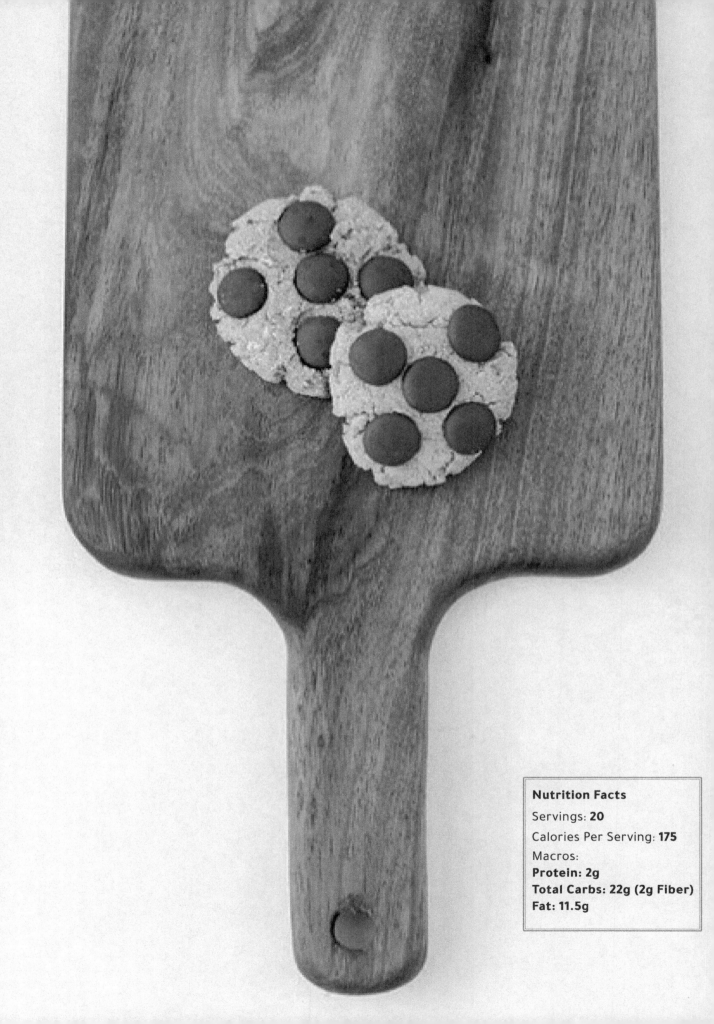

Quinoa Chocolate Chip Cookies

A healthy twist on my Mom's old chocolate chip cookie recipe! This, hands down, is the BEST gluten free chocolate chip cookie recipe you'll ever eat! Made with quinoa flour and coconut oil, these healthy gluten free, chocolate chip cookies will surprise you with incredible flavor and chewy texture. Easy to make and, best of all, you'd never know they're gluten free or made without butter! A cookie you can feel good about!

Ingredients

2 cups .... quinoa flour	2 .... eggs
1 tsp .... baking soda	2 tsp .... vanilla extract
1/2 tsp ...... salt	1 cup .... sugar free chocolate chips
2/3 cup ..... coconut oil, melted and cooled	1 tsp .... salt
1 1/3 cup .... monk fruit sweeter	

Preparation

1. Preheat oven to 350 F. Add quinoa flour to a large baking pan. Bake quinoa flour for 9-10 minutes. This is known as 'toasting' the quinoa flour and will help get rid of any bitterness. It's totally worth it as these cookies are so good! Once done toasting, transfer quinoa flour to a bowl to cool off for 5 minutes. Keep heat in oven.

2. In the large bowl, whisk together quinoa flour, baking soda, and salt; set aside.

3. In a separate large bowl, mix together melted and cooled coconut oil and sweetener until smooth. Add in eggs and vanilla and beat again until smooth and creamy.

4. Add in dry ingredients and mix together until combined and a dough forms. Fold in chocolate chips or chocolate chunks.

5. Roll dough into 1 inch balls and place on cookie sheet leaving 2 inches apart. Bake 8-11 minutes or until edges just being to turn a golden brown. Do not over bake; we don't want crispy cookies here! If you noticed that your cookies are baking super flat, then you may want to chill your dough for 10-20 minutes.

6. Remove from oven and let cool at least 5 minutes on baking sheet. The cookies will need to set and will be a little fragile at first so you have to be a little patient for the edges to harden a bit before removing them. This will test your patience and willpower HA!

7. Once the edges and bottom harden a bit, transfer to wire rack to finish cooling. Makes 20 cookies. Feel free to double the recipe if you want more.

Black Bean Brownies

This is a great way to use leftover sweet potatoes & black beans. The beans and whey protein powder pack in the protein and fiber, the potato adds beta carotene and a hint of sweetness, the coconut oil is full of healthy fats and the cocoa gives this recipe a boost of antioxidants. A great healthy treat, mid-day power snack or post workout recovery! If I'm having a sweet craving I'll enjoy these as my source of carbs for lunch.

Ingredients

1 1/2 cup....	black beans, organic, canned, drained , low-sodium
1/2 cup	sweet potato, cooked, mashed
2 tbsp	coconut oil
3/4 cup	whey protein powder, unflavored or chocolate
2 tbsp	monk fruit sweetener
1 1/2 tsp	vanilla extract

3/4 cup	gluten free flour mix
1/2 cup	cocoa, unsweetened
1/4 tsp	salt
1/2 cup	walnuts, chopped
1/2 cup	applesauce, unsweetened
1 tsp	baking powder
4	dates, pitted

Preparation

1. Preheat oven to 350 degree F. Lightly oil an 8" x 8" glass baking dish.

2. In the bowl of a food processor, combine black beans, sweet potatoes, coconut oil, dates, applesauce & vanilla. Puree.

3. In large bowl, sift flour, cocoa, baking powder & salt. Stir in wet ingredients to blend well; batter will be thick. Taste & adjust sweetening; if you prefer it sweeter add more monk fruit sweetener. Stir in walnuts.

4. Transfer batter to prepared baking dish & bake until set (approx. 40 minutes). Let cool then carefully turn out of the pan. Cut into 12 squares & serve.

Nutrition Facts

Servings: **12**
Calories Per Serving: **215**
Macros:
Protein: 10g
Total Carbs: 39g (6g Fiber)
Fat: 6g

RyFit Tip:
For a lower carb, higher fat option substitute a fat-based flour mix with blend of almond and coconut.

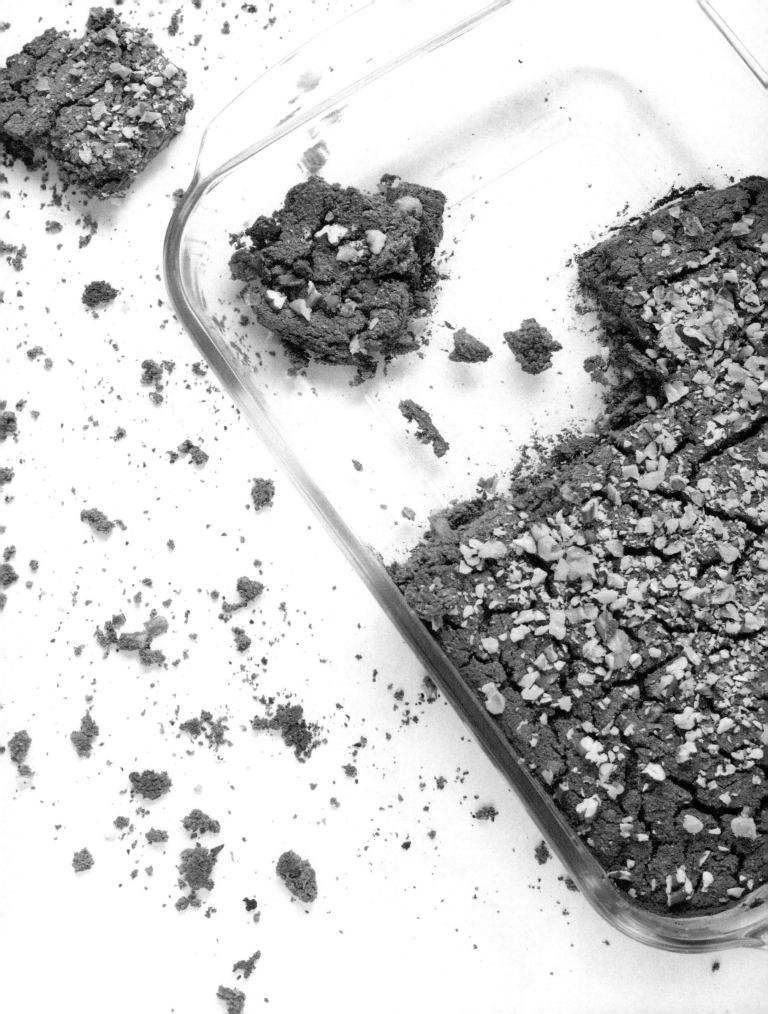

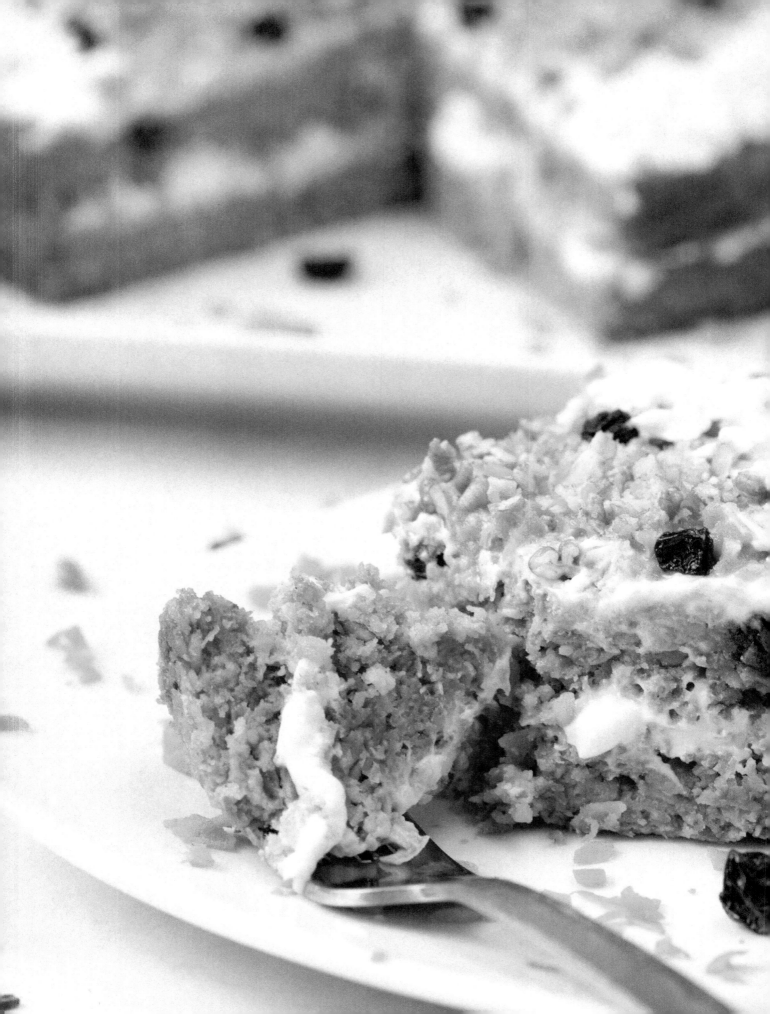

Vegan Carrot Cake

The BEST healthy carrot cake recipe you'll ever taste. Moist, cinnamon-spiced, and slathered in healthy frosting, it's perfect for celebrations (our motto is: everyday is a celebration!). Using applesauce, you can actually veganize carrot cake relatively easily. Along with the shredded carrots, it adds the perfect amount of moisture to eliminate the need for eggs or other unconventional ingredients.

Ingredients

1 cup .... carrot, shredded, packed

1/2 cup ...... applesauce, no sugar added

1/4 cup ...... coconut oil

2 tsp .... apple cider vinegar

2 tsp .... vanilla extract

1 1/2 tsp .... cinnamon

1 1/2 cups .. oat flour

3/4 tsp ...... salt

1/2 tsp ...... baking soda

1/4 cup ...... monk fruit sweetener

Preparation

1. Preheat oven to 350 F. Grease and line an 8-inch square or round pan with parchment. (If doubling the recipe, use two 8-inch pans or one 9x13.)

2. In a mixing bowl, whisk together the first 5 ingredients and let sit for at least 10 minutes or refrigerate overnight. Stir in all remaining ingredients. Optional add ins: handful shredded, raisins, unsweetened coconut, crushed walnuts or pecans. Try crushed pineapple instead of applesauce.

3. Pour into the pan, and smooth down. Bake 30 minutes or until a toothpick inserted into the cake comes out clean. If you can wait, I like to loosely cover once cool and let it sit overnight, because the cake tastes sweeter and has a lighter texture the next day! Leftovers can then be refrigerated 3-4 days or sliced and frozen. For a double layer cake or to fill a 9x13 pan, simply double all ingredients. Icing - use my protein cream cheese icing!

Nutrition Facts

Servings: **12**

Calories Per Serving: **215**

Macros:

Protein: 10g

Total Carbs: 39g (6g Fiber)

Fat: 6g

RyFit Tip:
Grate your carrots finely. Finely grated carrots meld seamlessly into the cake, while larger pieces leave a chunkier texture. For tender, cohesive cake slices, grate the carrots on the small holes of a box grater or on the smallest setting of the grating attachment on your food processor.
Don't overmix! This rule applies to baked goods across the board. Mix your batter until just combined, not any longer, or your cake will be dense.

Guilt-free Avocado Chocolate Pudding

This creamy avocado-based recipe is a healthy twist on a classic chocolate pudding. Full of healthy, satisfying fats and packed with fiber to reduce the total carbs - a rich, healthy dessert for anytime you have a chocolate craving (hello PMS!). Whip it up in under 5 minutes! I know it's going to be one of your favorites.

Ingredients

2.............. medium ripe avocado

4 tbsp....... cocoa powder, unsweetened

1/4 cup...... sugar free maple syrup

4 tbsp....... coconut milk, full fat

1/4 cup...... dark chocolate or chocolate chips, no sugar added

1/2 tsp ...... vanilla extract

1/8 tsp ...... salt

Preparation

1. Melt the dark chocolate and pour into all ingredients. Puree by hand or in a food processor until you get a fluffy and smooth pudding. Store in the fridge for 10 minutes before serving.

Nutrition Facts

Servings: **2**

Calories Per Serving: **325**

Macros:

Protein: 4.5g

Total Carbs: 33g (10.5g Fiber)

Fat: 29g

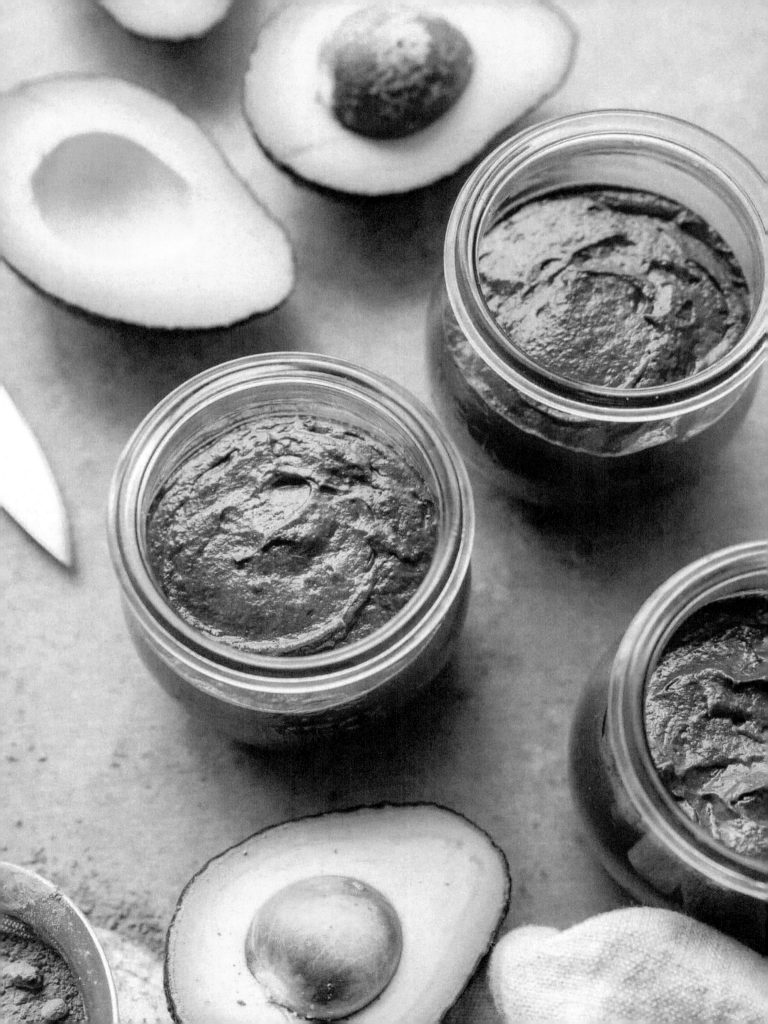

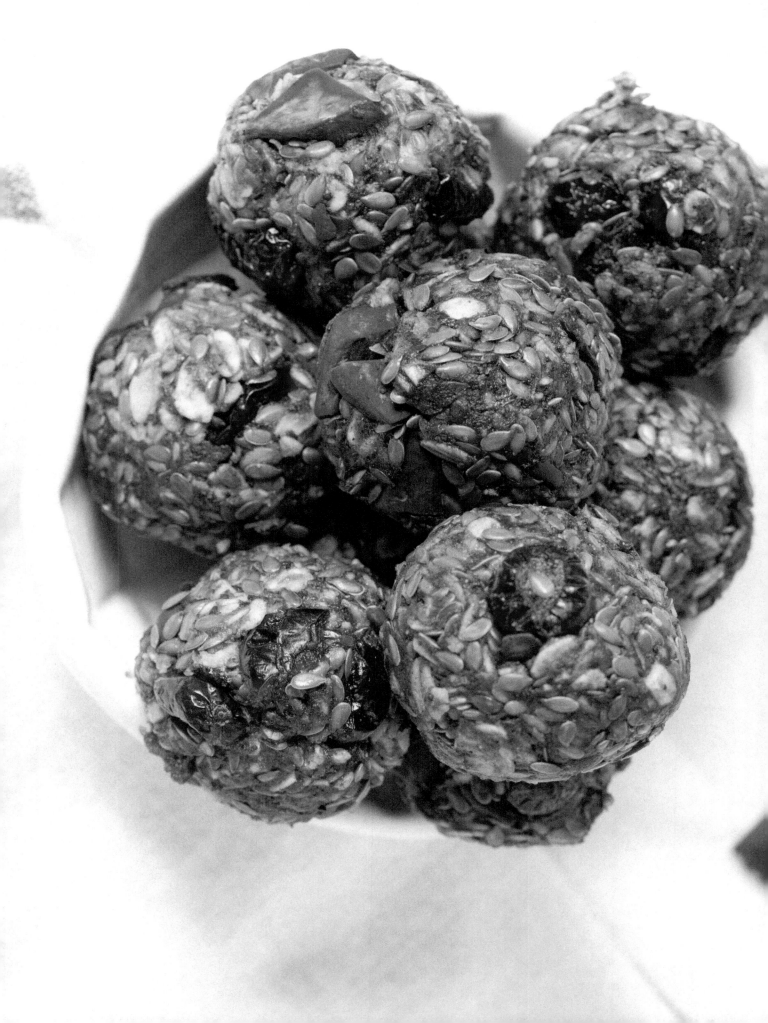

No Bake Protein CoffeeBites

This recipe contains 12g of fiber and is a great source of energy before a workout or perfect for a mid-morning pick-me up! Make extra and freeze them or make them child-friendly by kicking out the coffee beans.

Ingredients

1 cup .... gluten free oats

3/4 cup ..... whey protein powder

1/2 cup ...... flaxseed, ground

1 1/2 tbsp... coffee beans, fresh ground

1 cup .... almond butter, natural creamy

1 tbsp .... coconut oil

1/8 cup ...... unsweetened dairy free milk

1/4 cup ..... sugar free maple syrup

1 tsp .... vanilla extract

1/4 cup ...... chocolate chips or dark chocolate chunks, no sugar added

1 /4 cup ..... dried goji berries (optional)

Preparation

1. Stir oats, flaxseed, protein powder and coffee granules together in a medium bowl until thoroughly mixed, then add almond butter, coconut oil, syrup, milk and vanilla. Once combined well, fold in chocolate and goji berries. Stir well.

2. Chill in the refrigerator for 20 minutes. Once chilled, roll into balls of whatever size you would like, I usually make 10-12 balls. Store in an airtight container and keep in the fridge for up to 1 week...if they last that long!

Nutrition Facts
Servings: **10**
Calories Per Serving: **234**
Macros:
Protein: 5g
Total Carbs: 17g (2g Fiber)
Fat: 12g

RyFit Tip:
Peanut butter also works in place of the almond butter, however both MUST be creamy, and preferably store bought jars. While I love my self ground nut butters, they are much too dry for this recipe. When I say coffee grounds I mean take fresh beans, grind them, and use those grounds in the recipe. DO NOT brew them, and make sure your coffee is FRESH, old coffee will result in minimal coffee flavor. Also, the finer the grind of your coffee beans, the better the texture will be. If your coffee is too coarse you risk developing a cat-like sandpaper tongue. Yuck!

Vanilla Berry Protein Cheesecake

This is the most delicious, calorie-wise, satisfying protein cheesecake you'll ever have. It's calorie-smart, low in fat, moderate in carbs and it's packed with protein. Arrowroot powder is used as a more nutritious option than refined corn starch and if you're wanting lower carbs you can modify it easily by removing the crust and eating it like a pudding.

Ingredients

Filling

- 1 1/2 cups... whey protein powder, plain or vanilla
- 2 cups....... Greek yogurt, 0% plain
- 8 oz.......... cream cheese, fat free
- 1.............. egg white
- 3 tsp......... vanilla extract
- 4.5 tsp...... arrowroot powder
- 1 tbsp .... monk fruit sweetener

Crust

- 1 cup .... whey protein powder, plain or vanilla
- 1.5 cups..... graham cracker crumbs
- 5 tbsp .... unsweetened vegan milk
- 1 tbsp .... coconut oil

Preparation

1. Preheat oven to 300 degrees F. Spray 8x8 pan with olive or coconut oil spray.

2. Combine all the crust ingredients, form into dough and press tight into the pan. Bake the crust for 15 minutes.

3. Combine yogurt and cream cheese in a blender or food processor until smooth. Add egg white, vanilla extract, vanilla ice cream whey and arrowroot powder and mix again. Set aside.

4. When crust is cooled spread filling on top and bake for an additional 30 minutes.

5. Once cooked, chill in refrigerator for 4 hours and then top with fresh berries.

Nutrition Facts
Servings: **6**
Calories Per Serving: **145**
Macros:
Protein: 29g
Total Carbs: 22g (7g Fiber)
Fat: 3g

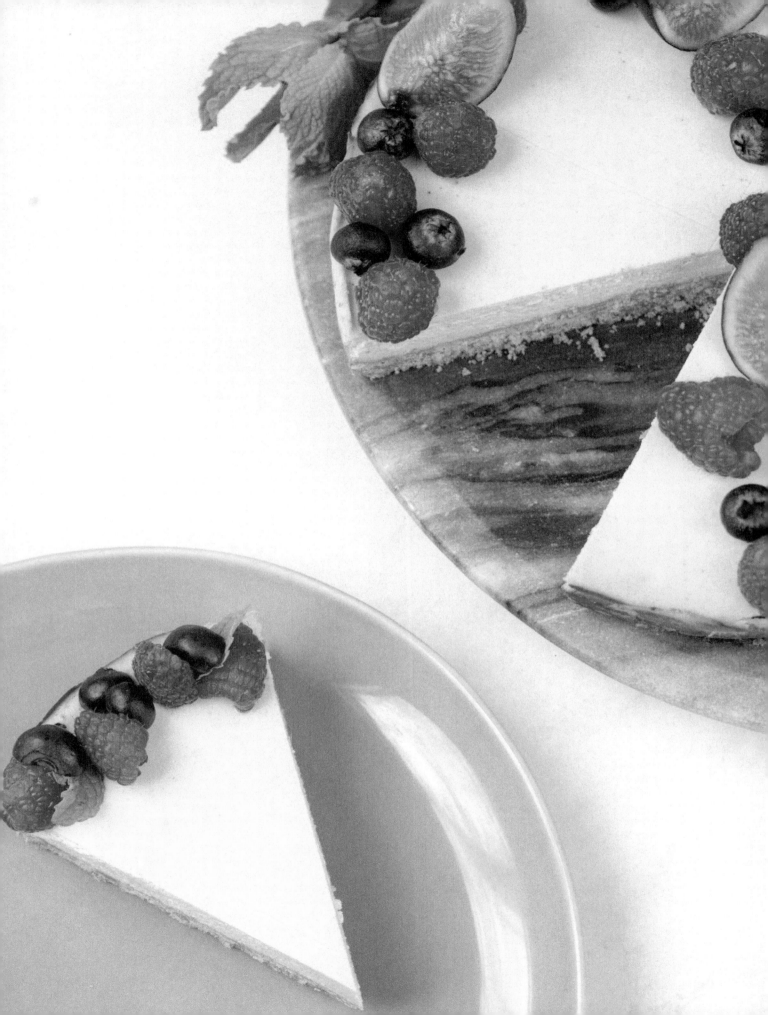

FIT COCKTAILS

We don't drink our calories

Until now! Now, I'm not promoting drinking alcohol regularly however I am an advocate for living a balanced lifestyle. And who doesn't love to enjoy a drink or two on occasion?! The word 'moderation' becomes key here. When choosing a 'healthier' alcoholic drink you want to opt for a red wine or a low sugar cocktail like the recipes I'm sharing with you in this chapter. These cocktails are all close to 100 calories and they're sugar free so you can avoid the hangover and won't blow your health and fitness goals.

Skinny Margarita

Ingredients

1 oz .... tequila

3 tbsp .... lime juice, freshly squeezed

1.5 tbsp ..... orange juice, freshly squeezed

1-2 tsp .... monk fruit simple syrup or
monk fruit drops (see page 356)

Preparation

1. Shake all ingredients over ice or blend for frozen version. Salt the rim of your glass (optional). Garnish with lime.

Magic Mojito

Ingredients

1 oz	....	rum	
12	....	mint leaves, fresh	
3 tbsp	....	lime juice, freshly squeezed	

7 oz .... mineral water

1–2 tsp .... monk fruit simple syrup or monk fruit drops (see page 356)

Preparation

1. Muddle the mint, lime and monk fruit in a glass. Add remaining ingredients and stir. I also love this with half mineral water and half coconut water.
Garnish with a lime.

Orange Spritzer

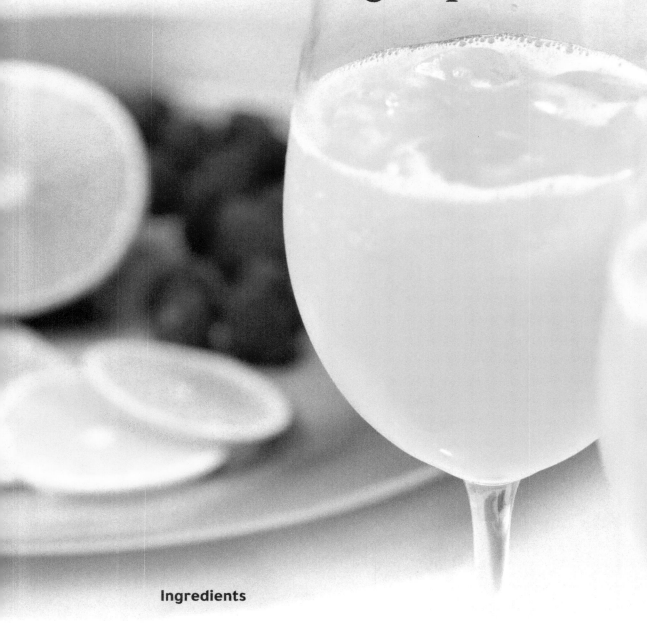

Ingredients

2 oz .... red wine

1/4 cup ...... orange juice, freshly squeezed

2 oz .... mineral water

1/2 cup ...... ice

Dash of cardamom or orange bitters

*optional but recommended

Preparation

1. Add red wine, orange juice and mineral water over ice.
Stir. Add in optional bitters and garish with an orange.

Berry Coconut Bliss

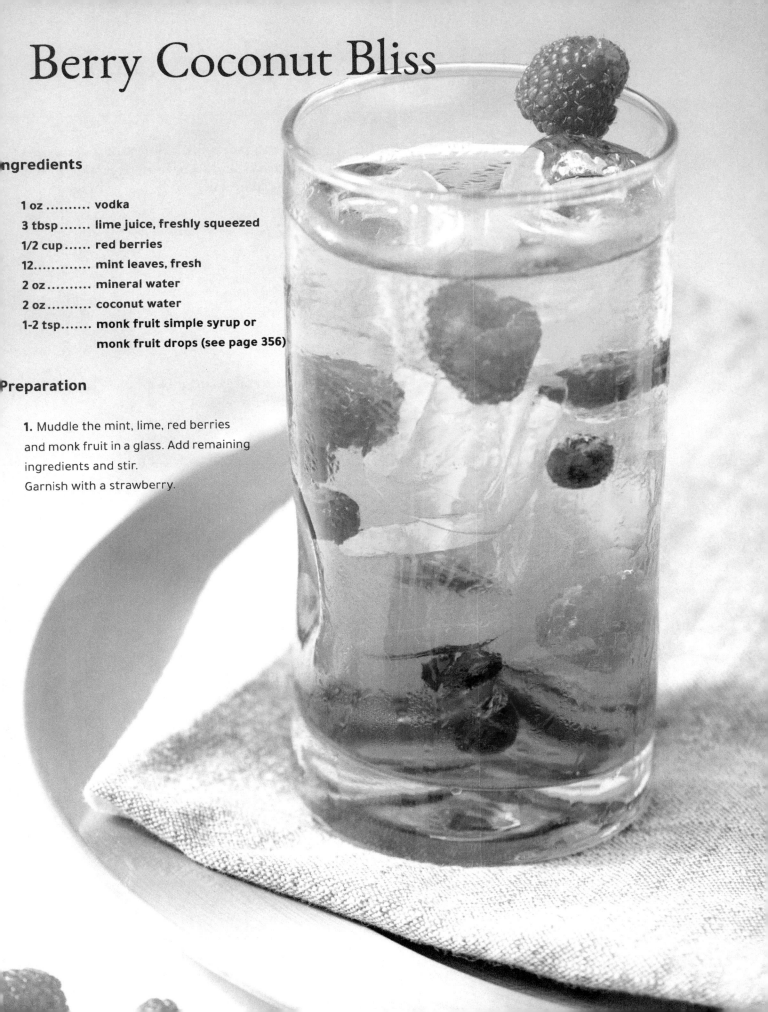

Ingredients

1 oz	vodka
3 tbsp	lime juice, freshly squeezed
1/2 cup	red berries
12	mint leaves, fresh
2 oz	mineral water
2 oz	coconut water
1-2 tsp	monk fruit simple syrup or monk fruit drops (see page 356)

Preparation

1. Muddle the mint, lime, red berries and monk fruit in a glass. Add remaining ingredients and stir. Garnish with a strawberry.

Monk Fruit Simple Syrup

Your own home-made, healthy 'simple syrup' - hello no sugar, carbs, calories or aftertaste (like you have with stevia)! It's perfect for all kinds of drinks and something I pack with me when I head out for a night on the town.

Ingredients

1 cup .... water
1/2 cup ...... granulated monk fruit

Preparation

1. Add water and monk fruit to a small saucepan and bring to a boil over medium/high heat. Stir regularly. Note - try to find pure monk fruit sweetener. If you can't find this then choose the blend with allulose which will dissolve better than erythritol and won't likely leave you bloated.

2. When the monk fruit sweetener has dissolved and the water is clear, remove and allow it to cool to room temperature. Transfer to an airtight container and store in the fridge for up to two weeks.

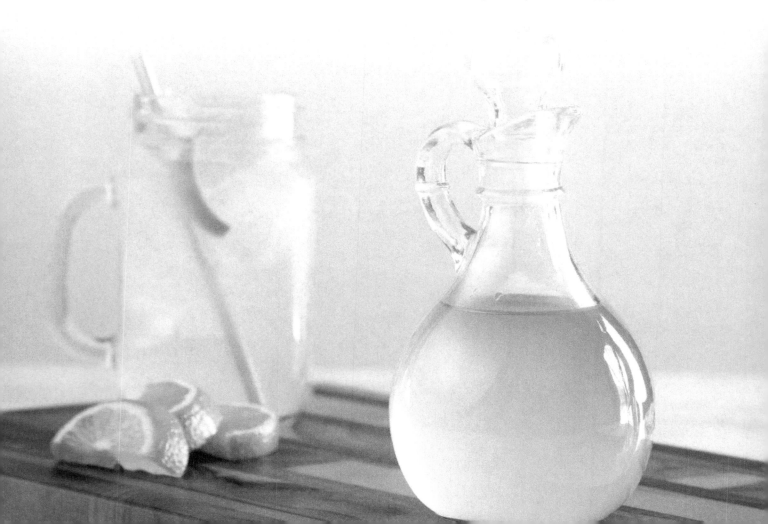

Ginger Kombucha Mule

Ingredients

1/2 cup	......	crushed ice
1 tbsp	....	freshly squeezed lime juice
1 ounce	.....	vodka
4 ounces	...	ginger-flavored kombucha
1 tsp	....	monk fruit simple syrup
		or monk fruit drops (see page 356)

For garnish:

Lime wedge, mint sprig, and/or slice of granny smith apple.

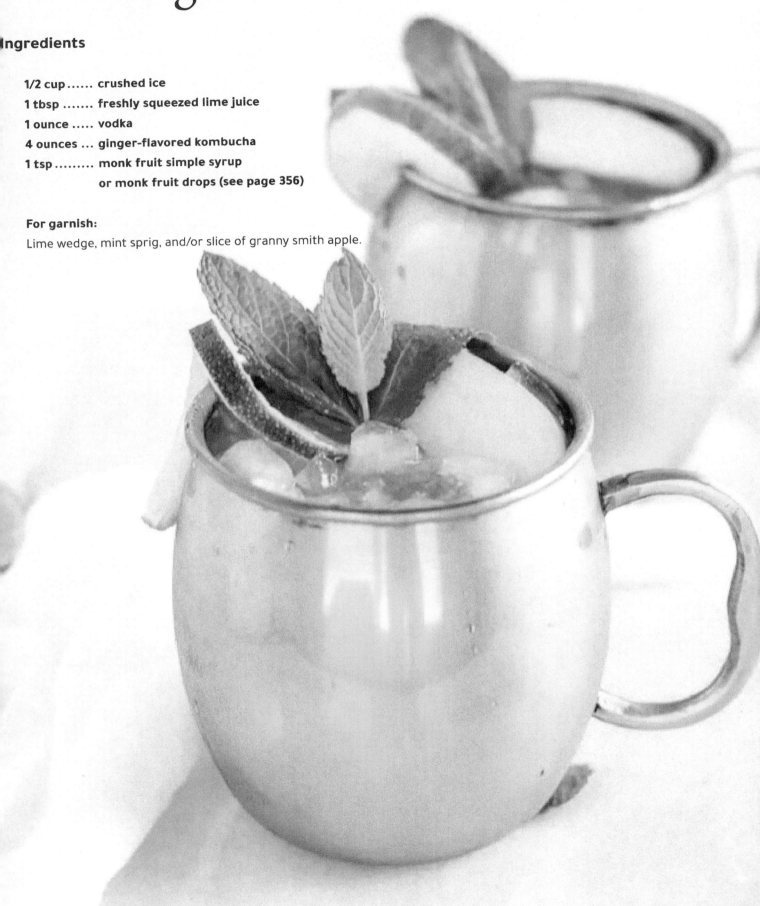

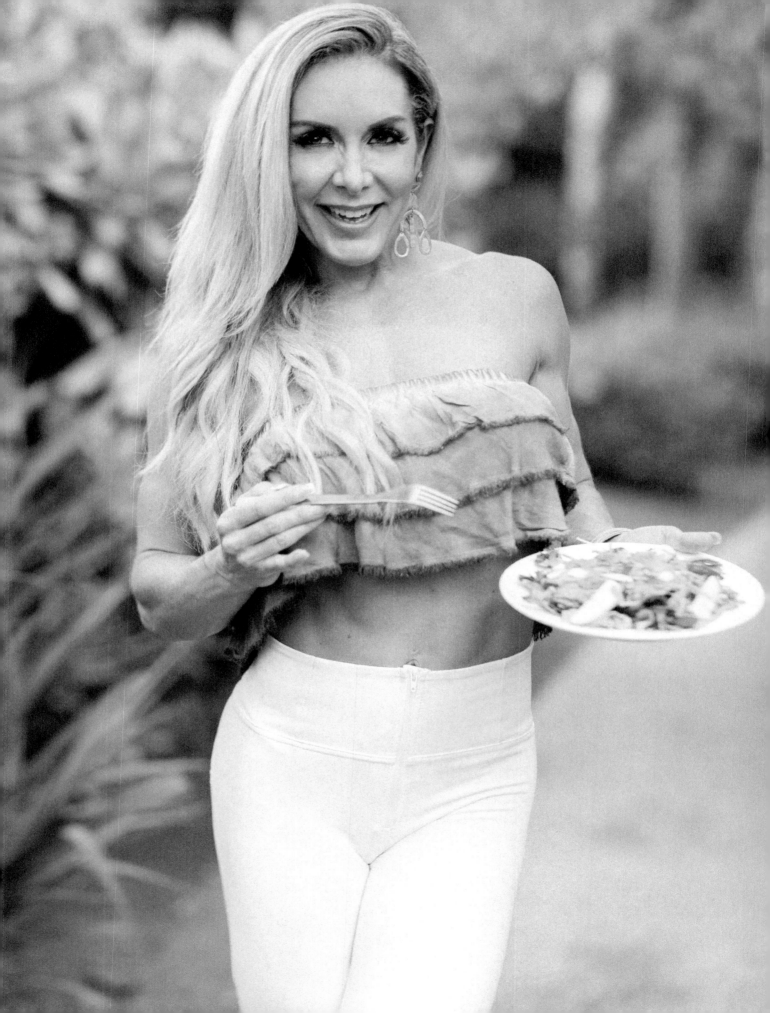

Metric Conversions
COMMON KITCHEN MEASUREMENTS

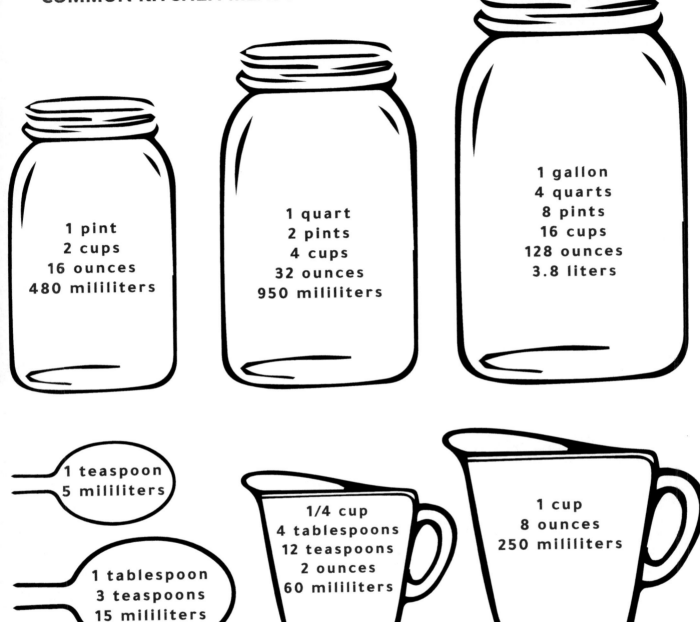

1 pint
2 cups
16 ounces
480 mililiters

1 quart
2 pints
4 cups
32 ounces
950 mililiters

1 gallon
4 quarts
8 pints
16 cups
128 ounces
3.8 liters

1 teaspoon
5 mililiters

1 tablespoon
3 teaspoons
15 mililiters

1/4 cup
4 tablespoons
12 teaspoons
2 ounces
60 mililiters

1 cup
8 ounces
250 mililiters

Temperature Conversions
Fahrenheit to Celsius (°F to °C)

500°F = 260°C   400°F = 205°C   300°F = 150°C
475°F = 245°C   375°F = 190°C   275°F = 135°C
450°F = 235°C   350°F = 180°C   250°F = 120°C
425°F = 220°C   325°F = 160°C   225°F = 110°C

Acknowledgments

'How To Eat' has been a labor of love. Over the past ten years I've had the great privilege of working with some very special people, and I can confidently say that this book wouldn't be possible if it wasn't for my 'dream team'. I'm forever grateful for the amazing talent, creativity and dedication that each of these people brought to this project.

MARCELO VAZQUEZ

Marcelo is the real VIP. My partner in life and in the kitchen, words can not convey how thankful I am for his unwavering support. He's been a huge contributor with recipe development - I'm the nutritionist and he's got the savvy kitchen skills. We've spent countless hours together, meticulously crafting the recipes In this book to perfection. Through the high times and hard times, he's continued to support me and never let me settle for less than I can achieve. This is 'our' Book, my love!

SHARIF KHALLADI

Sharif is my business mentor, digital marketing master, thought creator, fellow super-parent and dear friend; and he is one of the most influential people in my life. We started working together on this book a decade ago (when it was going to be a small recipe book not a 375 page book with recipes). When the book went on hold, as I pursued my quest to be the top-ranked fitness athlete in the world, he helped me build my online business into the empire that it is today. He's always believed in me; seen my potential and challenged me to think bigger. It's a great privilege to share space with him as his ideas are creative, outside the box and incredible valuable to me. He has had a tremendous impact on my life and I am so thankful for his wisdom, guidance and most of all, his friendship, over all these years.

VICTOR VAZQUEZ

I'm so lucky to have a bright web pro, marketing guru and awesome human on the back end of my business. 'Super V' has always got my back and he makes me smile. He's juggled the many moving parts of this project, while staying attentive and organized. He's wise beyond his years and I love picking his brain on the most recent marketing and sales strategies.

SUSAN VASCONCELOS

My graphics designer extraordinaire and vision creator! Sooz brought this book to life, finessing her way through hundreds of pages of text, details and folders full of images like a true pro. Because she is a pro! She totally gets me, even when I can't express myself creatively (my artistic muscle is pretty weak!), and she always blows me away with her creations. It's difficult to exceed my expectations, and she does it daily. Her sense of humor brightened the challenging days and I value her professionalism and design skills beyond words. We started this journey together over a decade ago and here we are now creating a book. I can't wait to see what we achieve in the next decade together! So thankful for you Susan.